KU-004-291

Multiple Choice Questions in Clinical Pharmacology

Second edition

Timothy GK Mant BSc, FFPM, FRCP
Medical Director,
Guy's Drug Research Unit, Guy's Hospital, London, UK

Lionel D Lewis MA, MD, FRCP
Associate Professor of Medicine and Pharmacology & Toxicology
Dartmouth Medical School and
Dartmouth-Hitchcock Medical Center,
Lebanon, NH, USA

James M Ritter MA, DPhil, FRCP
Professor of Clinical Pharmacology,
Guy's, King's and St Thomas's Medical Schools,
Guy's and St Thomas's NHS Hospital Trust,
London, UK

ARNOLD

A member of the Hodder Headline Group
LONDON   NEW YORK   NEW DELHI

First published in Great Britain in 1995
Second edition published in 2000 by Arnold.
A member of the Hodder Headline Group,
338 Euston Road, London NW1 3BH

Distributed in the United States of America by
Oxford University Press, Inc.,
198 Madison Avenue,
New York, NY 10016.
Oxford is a registered trademark of Oxford University Press

© 2001 Timothy G.K. Mant, Lionel D. Lewis and James M. Ritter

All rights reserved. No part of this publication may be reproduced or transmitted
in any form or by any means, electronically or mechanically, including
photocopying, recording or any information storage or retrieval system, without
either prior permission in writing from the publisher or a licence permitting
restricted copying. In the United Kingdom such licences are issued by the
Copyright Licensing Agency: 90 Tottenham Court Road, London W1P 9HE.

Whilst the advice and information in this book is believed to be true and
accurate at the date of going to press, neither the authors nor the publisher can
accept any legal responsibility for any errors or omissions that may be made. In
particular (but without limiting the generality of the preceding disclaimer) every
effort has been made to check drug dosages; however, it is still possible that
errors have been missed. Furthermore, dosage schedules are constantly being
revised and new side effects recognized. For these reasons the reader is strongly
urged to consult the drug companies' printed instructions before administering
any of the drugs recommended in this book.

British Library Cataloguing in Publication Data
A catalogue record for this book is available from the British Library

Library of Congress Cataloging-in-Publication Data
A catalog record for this book is available from the Library of Congress

ISBN 0 340 76295 0

Typeset in 9/11pt Legacy Serif by Phoenix Photosetting, Chatham, Kent
Printed and bound in Great Britain by MPG Books Ltd, Bodmin, Cornwall

What do you think about this book? Or any other Arnold title?
Please send your comments to feedback.arnold@hodder.co.uk

Contents

Introduction

Multiple choice questions are now ubiquitous in the final medical examinations. They provide a rapid method for testing a wide range of knowledge and marking is objective. The authors, all practising physicians who have taught clinical pharmacology and therapeutics for many years, have based this book around the fourth edition of *Textbook of Clinical Pharmacology* not only to prepare students for their exams but also to emphasize those principles and facts which are the key to safe and effective prescribing.

The answers are related to the relevant section in *Textbook of Clinical Pharmacology (TCP)*. In addition there are brief annotations on each question.

Although this book can "stand alone", we hope students will read a section of the main textbook and then reinforce and revise their knowledge by self-testing using the multiple choice questions (MCQ) book. At the end of the book is a practice examination of 60 questions. It covers the spectrum of topics that may be encountered in a final MB examination. We suggest that students use this as a "practice run" after finishing their revision of the subject as a whole. It is best to do it "blind" at one sitting lasting not more than 90 minutes. Many MCQ exams mark +2 for a correct response, 0 for no response and –1 for an incorrect response. Fifty per cent is the pass mark for the exam at the end of the book (i.e. 300/600 possible marks).

We thank the generations of students who have provided critical feedback, Dr Dipti Amin for her review of the questions and answers and Gill Manners for her word processing skills and patience.

CHAPTER ONE

General Principles

1 The following drugs have been correctly paired with a measure of their pharmacodynamic effect:

   (a) Warfarin – prolongation of prothrombin time
   (b) Insulin – reduction in blood glucose
   (c) Atenolol – reduction in exercise-induced tachycardia
   (d) Morphine – pupil dilation
   (e) Omeprazole – inhibition of gastric acid secretion

2 The following drugs exert their effects by combining with receptors and mimicking the effects of the natural mediator (i.e. are agonists):

   (a) Tamoxifen
   (b) Salbutamol
   (c) Morphine
   (d) Cetirizine
   (e) Captopril

3 The following drugs exert their principal effects by enzyme inhibition:

   (a) Pyridostigmine
   (b) Atropine
   (c) Amlodipine
   (d) Digoxin
   (e) Selegiline

4 The following drugs are reversible competitive antagonists:

   (a) Suxamethonium
   (b) Chlorpheniramine
   (c) Ranitidine
   (d) Phenoxybenzamine
   (e) Naloxone

1 (a) **True**   Pharmacodynamics is the study of the effects of drugs on
   (b) **True**   biological processes. One of the pharmacodynamic effects
   (c) **True**   of morphine is pupil constriction
   (d) **False**
   (e) **True**

2 (a) **False** – Tamoxifen is an anti-estrogen used in breast cancer
   (b) **True**   – Salbutamol is a β-agonist. It is relatively selective for β_2
                    effects (bronchodilation) but at higher doses β_1 effects
                    (tachycardia and tremor) also occur
   (c) **True**   – Morphine mimics the endogenous encephalins
   (d) **False** – Cetirizine is an antihistamine (H_1-blocker)
   (e) **False** – Captopril is an angiotensin-converting enzyme inhibitor

3 (a) **True**   – Pyridostigmine is an inhibitor of acetylcholinesterase and is
                    used in myasthenia gravis
   (b) **False** – Atropine blocks muscarinic receptors
   (c) **False** – Amlodipine is a calcium channel blocker
   (d) **True**   – Digoxin inhibits Na^+/K^+ adenosine triphosphatase (ATPase)
   (e) **True**   – Selegiline is an MAO-B inhibitor used in Parkinson's disease

4 (a) **False** – Suxamethonium is an agonist that causes a seemingly
                    paradoxical inhibitory effect (neuromuscular blockade) by
                    causing long-lasting depolarization of the neuromuscular
                    junction
   (b) **True**   – Chlorpheniramine is a histamine (H_1) antagonist
   (c) **True**   – Ranitidine is a histamine (H_2) antagonist
   (d) **False** – Phenoxybenzamine is an irreversible α-receptor antagonist
   (e) **True**   – Naloxone is a competitive antagonist at the morphine
                    μ-receptor

5 The following drugs are partial agonists:

(a) Isoprenaline
(b) Morphine
(c) Naloxone
(d) Buprenorphine
(e) Oxprenolol

6 The following drugs cause their effects via non-receptor mechanisms:

(a) Magnesium trisilicate
(b) Mannitol
(c) Ispaghula
(d) Dimercaprol
(e) Sumatriptan

7 The pharmacokinetic "half-life" of the following drugs resembles their pharmacodynamic "half-life":

(a) Salbutamol
(b) Phenelzine
(c) Dobutamine
(d) Omeprazole
(e) Cyclophosphamide

8 The plasma clearance of a drug:

(a) Is the volume of plasma from which the drug is totally eliminated per unit time
(b) Is equal to the administration rate at steady state divided by the steady state plasma concentration
(c) Is a better measure of the efficiency of drug elimination than elimination half-life
(d) Does not include elimination by hepatic metabolism
(e) May be affected by renal function

GENERAL PRINCIPLES

5 (a) **False**   Partial agonists combine with receptors but are incapable of
  (b) **False**   eliciting a maximal response whatever their concentration
  (c) **False**
  (d) **True**   – Buprenorphine is a partial agonist at the opiate µ-receptor
  (e) **True**   – Oxprenolol is a partial agonist at the β-adrenoceptor

6 (a) **True**   – Magnesium trisilicate is an antacid which neutralizes gastric
             acid
  (b) **True**   – Mannitol is an osmotic diuretic
  (c) **True**   – Ispaghula is a bulk laxative
  (d) **True**   – Dimercaprol is a chelating agent used in heavy metal
             poisoning
  (e) **False** – Sumatriptan is a $5HT_{1D}$ agonist used in migraine

7 (a) **True**   The magnitude of pharmacological effect usually depends
  (b) **False** directly on the concentration of drug (or active metabolites) in
  (c) **True**   the vicinity of their receptors. However, some drugs form
  (d) **False** irreversible bonds at their sites of action so their effects
  (e) **False** outlast their presence at these sites (e.g. alkylating agents).

8 (a) **True**   Clearance and not half-life should be used as a measure of
  (b) **True**   the efficiency of drug elimination. Clearance is independent
  (c) **True**   of volume of distribution.
  (d) **False**
  (e) **True**

9 For a drug that obeys first order (linear) kinetics and fits a one-compartment model of elimination:

(a) Its rate of elimination is proportional to its plasma concentration
(b) Following cessation of an intravenous infusion the plasma concentration declines exponentially
(c) The half-life is proportional to the dose
(d) The half-life is unaffected by renal function
(e) The composition of drug products excreted is independent of the dose

10 The apparent volume of distribution:

(a) Can be greater than the total body volume
(b) Is approximately 3 litres for most drugs in adults
(c) Is influenced by a drug's lipid solubility
(d) A large value indicates that a drug will be efficiently eliminated by hemodialysis
(e) Determines the peak plasma concentration after a bolus intravenous dose

9 (a) **True** Although the one compartment model is an oversimplification,
  (b) **True** once absorption and distribution are complete many drugs
  (c) **False** do obey first order elimination kinetics: See Fig. 1 below.
  (d) **False**
  (e) **True**

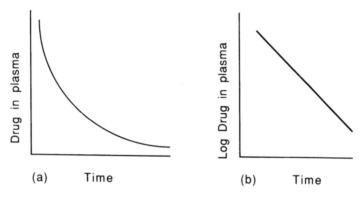

(a)   Time   (b)   Time

Fig. 1 One-compartment model. Plasma concentration–time curve following a bolus dose of drug plotted (a) arithmetically, or (b) semi-logarithmically. This drug fits a one-compartment model, i.e. its concentration falls exponentially with time

10 (a) **True** Volume of distribution = dose/C_0. C_0 is the plasma concentration
   (b) **False** at time zero calculated by extrapolation following a bolus
   (c) **True** intravenous injection. 3 litres is the approximate total plasma
   (d) **False** volume in an adult.
   (e) **True**

11 The following drugs have an elimination half-life less than 4 hours in a healthy adult:

   (a) Dopamine
   (b) Heparin
   (c) Amiodarone
   (d) Gentamicin
   (e) Diazepam

12 In repeated (multiple) dosing:

   (a) If the dosing interval is much greater than the half-life little if any accumulation occurs
   (b) It takes approximately five half-lives to reach 50% of the steady state concentration
   (c) If a drug is administered once every half-life once steady state is reached, the peak plasma concentration will be double the trough concentration
   (d) The use of a bolus loading dose reduces the time taken to reach steady state
   (e) In renal impairment the dosing interval should be increased when prescribing gentamicin

13 The following drugs obey non-linear (dose-dependent) elimination pharmacokinetics in therapeutic doses:

   (a) Salicylate
   (b) Heparin
   (c) Phenytoin
   (d) Ethanol
   (e) Cefuroxime

14 The following undergo enterohepatic recycling:

   (a) Estrogens
   (b) Cefuroxime
   (c) Rifampicin
   (d) Gentamicin
   (e) Ciprofloxacin

11 (a) **True** – Dopamine, 2 minutes
   (b) **True** – Heparin, 0.5–2.5 hours
   (c) **False** – Amiodarone, 28–45 days
   (d) **True** – Gentamicin, 2 hours
   (e) **False** – Diazepam, 20–50 hours

12 (a) **True**   It takes approximately three half-lives to reach 87.5% of
   (b) **False** steady state. After four half-lives it is 93.75% and after five
   (c) **True**   half-lives 96.9%.
   (d) **True**
   (e) **True**

13 (a) **True**   Implications of non-linear elimination kinetics include:
   (b) **True**   the time taken to eliminate 50% of a dose increases with
   (c) **True**   increasing dose i.e. half-life increases with dose; once the
   (d) **True**   drug elimination process is saturated, a relatively modest
   (e) **False** increase in dose dramatically increases the amount of drug in
                  the body.

14 (a) **True**   Enterohepatic recycling is when a drug is excreted into the
   (b) **False** bile, reabsorbed from the intestine and returned via the
   (c) **True**   portal system to the liver to be recycled.
   (d) **False**
   (e) **False**

15 The oral bioavailability of a drug:

  (a) Is a measure of the extent to which it enters the systemic circulation
  (b) May be influenced by changing the excipient from calcium sulfate to lactose
  (c) Is determined by comparing the area under the plasma concentration time curve (AUC) following oral and intravenous administration
  (d) May be reduced by hepatic enzyme induction
  (e) Two preparations of a drug may have similar bioavailability but have different peak concentrations

16 The following are examples of prodrugs:

  (a) Levodopa
  (b) Azathioprine
  (c) Benorilate
  (d) Sulfasalazine
  (e) Frusemide (furosemide)

17 The following oral drugs do not require absorption from the gut to exert a therapeutic effect:

  (a) Acarbose
  (b) Methionine
  (c) Colestyramine
  (d) Olsalazine
  (e) Vancomycin

18 Drug absorption following oral administration:

  (a) Is most commonly through passive diffusion
  (b) Occurs predominantly in the colon
  (c) Is usually complete within 60 minutes
  (d) Non-polar lipid-soluble drugs are absorbed more readily than polar water-soluble drugs
  (e) Peptides are well absorbed following oral administration

15 (a) **True**   See *Textbook of Clinical Pharmacology (TCP)*, Chapter 4,
   (b) **True**   pp. 26–28. Although the bioavailability of two preparations
   (c) **True**   may be the same, the kinetics can be very different as seen in
   (d) **True**   some immediate and slow release formulations.
   (e) **True**

16 (a) **True** – Levodopa → dopamine
   (b) **True** – Azathioprine → 6-mercaptopurine
   (c) **True** – Benorylate → paracetamol + aspirin
   (d) **True** – Sulfasalazine → aminosalicylate + sulfapyridine
   (e) **False**

17 (a) **True** – Acarbose is a competitive inhibitor of intestinal
           α-glucosidases
   (b) **False** – Methionine, an antidote to paracematol poisoning, acts not
           in the gastrointestinal tract but predominantly in the liver
           where it repletes glutathione which inactivates the toxic
           paracetamol metabolite
   (c) **True** – Colestyramine is a bile acid binding resin which indirectly
           lowers plasma low density lipoprotein (LDL) cholesterol
           hence it has a systemic effect without systemic drug
           absorption
   (d) **True** – Olsalazine delivers 5-aminosalicylate to the colon where it
           has a local action in inflammatory bowel disease
   (e) **True** – Vancomycin kills toxin producing *Clostridium difficile*, the
           cause of pseudomembranous colitis within the bowel

18 (a) **True**   Most oral drugs are absorbed by passive diffusion in the
   (b) **False**   small bowel. In general low molecular weight, high lipid
   (c) **False**   solubility and lack of charge encourage absorption. Most
   (d) **True**   peptides are broken down enzymatically.
   (e) **False**

19 The following drugs are absorbed predominantly through active transport systems:

(a) Paracetamol (acetaminophen)
(b) Phenytoin
(c) Levodopa
(d) Methyldopa
(e) Lithium

20 The systemic bioavailability of the following oral drugs is increased if taken in the fasting state:

(a) Oxytetracycline
(b) Ampicillin
(c) Levodopa
(d) Acetylsalicylic acid/salicylates
(e) Griseofulvin

21 The following drugs are usefully administered by the sublingual route:

(a) Digoxin
(b) Carbamazepine
(c) Captopril
(d) Buprenorphine
(e) Glyceryl trinitrate

22 The following drugs are usefully administered by the rectal route for their systemic effect:

(a) Indomethacin
(b) Sulfasalazine
(c) Metronidazole
(d) Glycerin
(e) Diazepam

19 (a) **False**   Active transport requires specific carrier-mediated energy
   (b) **False**   consuming mechanisms. Naturally occurring polar nutrients
   (c) **True**   and aliments including sugars, amino-acids and vitamins are
   (d) **True**   absorbed by active or facilitated transport mechanisms.
   (e) **True**   Drugs that are analogs of such molecules compete for
                    uptake. Further examples include methotrexate and
                    5-fluorouracil.

20 (a) **True**   Food and drink dilute the drug and can adsorb or otherwise
   (b) **True**   compete with it. Transient increases in hepatic blood flow
   (c) **False**   such as occur after a meal may result in greater availability of
   (d) **False**   drug by reducing presystemic hepatic metabolism.
   (e) **False**

21 (a) **False**   Sublingual administration can be an effective means of
   (b) **False**   causing systemic effects, and has potential advantages over
   (c) **False**   oral administration (i.e. when the drug is swallowed) for
   (d) **True**   drugs with pronounced presystemic metabolism, providing
   (e) **True**   direct and rapid access to the systemic circulation bypassing
                    intestine and liver. See *TCP*, Chapter 4, p. 31.

22 (a) **True**   – Rectal indomethacin administered at night is useful in
                    reducing early morning stiffness in rheumatoid arthritis
   (b) **False** – Rectal sulfasalazine is used for its local effect in
                    inflammatory bowel disease
   (c) **True**   – Rectal metronidazole is well absorbed (and much less
                    expensive than the intravenous preparation)
   (d) **False** – Glycerin suppositories exert a local effect to stimulate
                    defecation
   (e) **True**   – Rectal diazepam is used to control convulsions when venous
                    access is difficult (as may be the case in children)

23 The following drugs may be applied to the skin to produce systemic therapeutic effect:

(a) Glyceryl trinitrate
(b) Estradiol
(c) Lignocaine (lidocaine)
(d) Hydrocortisone
(e) Nicotine

24 Intramuscular injection:

(a) Rate of absorption is enhanced by exercise
(b) Rate of absorption is greater from the deltoid injection site than the gluteus maximus site
(c) If administered to the buttock should be in the upper outer quadrant
(d) Should usually be no greater than 0.5 mL
(e) Is an appropriate route of administration for the decanoate ester of fluphenazine

25 The following are commonly associated with phlebitis when given via the intravenous route:

(a) Erythromycin
(b) Hydrocortisone
(c) Diazepam
(d) 50% Glucose
(e) 5% Glucose

26 The following are metabolized in hepatic smooth endoplasmic reticulum:

(a) Levodopa
(b) Tyramine
(c) Theophylline
(d) Suxamethonium
(e) 6-Mercaptopurine

23 (a) **True** – Transdermal GTN is used in ischemic heart disease and is being investigated in premature labor
   (b) **True** – Transdermal estradiol is used for hormone replacement therapy in menopausal women
   (c) **False** – Local lignocaine is used for its local anesthetic action (e.g. for intravenous cannulation in children)
   (d) **False** – Topical hydrocortisone is used for a local anti-inflammatory action without the disadvantage of systemic corticosteroids
   (e) **True** – Nicotine is used to assist cigarette smokers to abstain

24 (a) **True** – Exercise and local massage increase the rate of absorption
   (b) **True** – Transport from the injection site is governed by muscle blood flow – deltoid > vastus lateralis > gluteus maximus
   (c) **True** – This avoids the risk of sciatic nerve palsy
   (d) **False** – Up to 5 mL is acceptable in the buttock
   (e) **True** – This depot preparation is slowly hydrolyzed in muscle to release active drug and is used to improve compliance in schizophrenic patients

25 (a) **True** – A macrolide antibiotic
   (b) **False**
   (c) **True** – An oily emulsion (Diazemuls™) reduces this complication
   (d) **True** – Used in hypoglycemic coma
   (e) **False**

26 (a) **False** – Levodopa is decarboxylated to dopamine in central neurons
   (b) **False** – Tyramine is metabolized by monoamine oxidase (MAO) in intestine, liver, kidney and nervous tissue. MAO is a mitochondrial enzyme
   (c) **True** – Theophylline is extensively metabolized by the CYP_{450} system
   (d) **False** – Suxamethonium is metabolized by plasma cholinesterase
   (e) **False** – Purines (e.g. 6-mercaptopurine) are metabolized by xanthine oxidase which is a non-microsomal enzyme

27 The following are substrates for cytochrome P_{450}:

(a) Procainamide
(b) Erythromycin
(c) Phenytoin
(d) Adrenaline (epinephrine)
(e) Warfarin

28 The following drugs are acetylated:

(a) Dapsone
(b) Cyclosporin
(c) Gentamicin
(d) Isoniazid
(e) Hydralazine

29 The following cause hepatic enzyme (microsomal cytochrome P_{450}) induction:

(a) Rifampicin
(b) Carbamazepine
(c) St John's wort
(d) Phenobarbitone
(e) Penicillin

27 (a) **False** – Procainamide is acetylated. Procainamide is used to treat ventricular arrhythmias

   (b) **True** – Erythromycin as well as being metabolized by cytochrome P_{450} enzymes inhibits the metabolism of other drugs subject to cytochrome P_{450} metabolism (e.g. warfarin, theophylline and terfenadine)

   (c) **True** – Phenytoin also induces cytochrome P_{450} enzymes

   (d) **False** – Adrenaline is a catecholamine and is metabolized by catechol-O-methyltransferase which is present in the cytosol

   (e) **True** – Warfarin has a narrow therapeutic index

28 (a) **True** – Dapsone is used in leprosy and dermatitis herpetiformis

   (b) **False** – Cyclosporin, an immunosuppressant, is metabolized by CYP_{450}

   (c) **False** – Gentamicin is eliminated unchanged by the kidney

   (d) **True** – Isoniazid is used to treat TB

   (e) **True** – Hydralazine is a vasodilator used as an adjunct to other treatment for hypertension. When used alone it causes tachycardia and fluid retention. It can cause an SLE-like syndrome which is more common in slow acetylators. An intravenous preparation is available to treat hypertensive crises in pregnancy

29 (a) **True** – Rifampicin is a broad spectrum antibiotic used in tuberculosis and Legionnaire's disease

   (b) **True** – Carbamazepine is an anticonvulsant

   (c) **True** – St John's wort, a herbal remedy, may be purchased without a prescription. It is a potent, broad spectrum CYP_{450} enzyme inducer

   (d) **True** – Phenobarbitone is an anticonvulsant

   (e) **False** – Penicillin is predominantly eliminated unchanged in the urine

Drug interactions secondary to hepatic enzyme induction and inhibition are clinically significant when there is a close correlation between plasma concentration and effect, and a steep dose response curve. Regular use of ethanol induces CYP_{450} metabolism but has minimal effect on its own metabolism, which is predominantly via cytoplasmic alcohol dehydrogenase.

30 The following inhibit cytochrome P_{450}:

(a) Fluvoxamine
(b) Grapefruit juice
(c) Digoxin
(d) Ketoconazole
(e) Ciprofloxacin

31 The following are subject to extensive presystemic metabolism:

(a) Chlorpheniramine
(b) Phenytoin
(c) Ciprofloxacin
(d) Morphine
(e) Verapamil

32 The following decrease the rate of gastric emptying:

(a) Myocardial infarction
(b) Migraine
(c) Myxedema
(d) Duodenal ulcer
(e) Metoclopramide

33 Cardiac failure:

(a) Reduces the bioavailability of thiazide diuretics
(b) Increases the volume of distribution of lignocaine (lidocaine)
(c) Has little effect on the volume of distribution of frusemide (furosemide)
(d) Decreases the terminal half-life of lignocaine (lidocaine)
(e) Decreases the terminal half-life of gentamicin

30 (a) **True** – Fluvoxamine, an antidepressant, is a selective serotonin reuptake inhibitor which inhibits the metabolism of theophylline and warfarin

   (b) **True** – Grapefruit containing products inhibit CYP_{450}, probably predominantly in the intestine

   (c) **False** – Digoxin is predominantly eliminated unchanged in the urine

   (d) **True** – Ketoconazole is an antifungal agent

   (e) **True** – Ciprofloxacin is a fluoroquinolone antibacterial drug

31 (a) **False**   Presystemic metabolism occurs in the gastrointestinal

   (b) **False**   mucosa and liver; presystemic (first pass) metabolism

   (c) **False**   necessitates high oral doses in comparison with the

   (d) **True**   intravenous dose.

   (e) **True**

32 (a) **True** – Pain decreases the rate of gastric emptying

   (b) **True**

   (c) **True**

   (d) **False**

   (e) **False** – Metoclopramide accelerates gastric emptying

33 (a) **True** – The absorption of thiazides is reduced by 30–40%

   (b) **False** – The volume of distribution of lignocaine is reduced probably because of decreased tissue perfusion

   (c) **True** – The distribution volume of frusemide is largely confined to the vascular compartment

   (d) **False** – Is prolonged predominantly due to decreased hepatic perfusion

   (e) **False** – Glomerular filtration is reduced in cardiac failure and hence the elimination half-life of gentamicin is prolonged (i.e. not decreased)

34 In severe renal failure:

(a) Gastric pH decreases
(b) The "therapeutic range" for phenytoin decreases
(c) Drug distribution to the brain is decreased
(d) Smaller maintenance doses of digoxin are required
(e) Inulin clearance gives a more accurate estimate of glomerular filtration rate than creatinine clearance

35 The following statements are correct:

(a) The kidneys receive approximately 20% of the cardiac output
(b) In healthy young adults approximately 130 mL/min of protein-free filtrate is formed at the glomeruli
(c) Non-protein bound drug of molecular weight < 66 000 passes into the filtrate
(d) Potentially saturable mechanisms for active secretion of both acids and bases exist in the proximal tubule
(e) Low lipid solubility favors tubular reabsorption

36 The following are actively secreted into the tubular fluid in the proximal segment:

(a) Inulin
(b) Probenecid
(c) Penicillin
(d) Para-aminohippuric acid (PAH)
(e) Cimetidine

37 The following drugs must be avoided in severe renal failure (glomerular filtration rate <10 mL/min):

(a) Prednisolone
(b) Amoxicillin
(c) Bumetanide
(d) Metformin
(e) Oxytetracycline

34 (a) **False** – Gastric pH increases
   (b) **True** – The ratio of unbound : bound phenytoin rises in renal failure. It is unbound drug which is active and the laboratory assay for phenytoin measures total blood concentration (bound and unbound)
   (c) **False** – The blood–brain barrier becomes functionally less of a barrier to drug distribution in severe renal failure. This may be the reason for the increased incidence of confusion associated with cimetidine in renal failure
   (d) **True** – The volume of distribution is decreased and renal clearance reduced
   (e) **True** – Inulin clearance is the "gold standard" measure of glomerular filtration rate

35 (a) **True**   The kidney is involved to some degree in the elimination of
   (b) **True**   virtually every drug or drug metabolite in man. High lipid
   (c) **True**   solubility and the unionized state favor reabsorption.
   (d) **True**
   (e) **False**

36 (a) **False**   Unlike glomerular filtration, tubular secretion can eliminate
   (b) **True**   drugs efficiently even if they are protein bound. For some
   (c) **True**   acidic drugs (e.g. benzylpenicillin) virtually all of the drug is
   (d) **True**   excreted by the organic acid transport mechanism.
   (e) **True**   Competition can occur (e.g. probenecid and penicillin).

37 (a) **False** – Prednisolone is a corticosteroid
   (b) **False** – Reduce dose; rashes more common
   (c) **False** – May need very high doses for any effect
   (d) **True** – Increased risk of lactic acidosis
   (a) **True** – Direct nephrotoxicity, anti-anabolic, increases blood urea

38 The following can impair renal function:

(a) Naproxen
(b) Ranitidine
(c) Iodine-containing contrast media
(d) Captopril
(e) Amphotericin B

39 The following drugs should be avoided in hepatic failure:

(a) Spironolactone
(b) Chlorpromazine
(c) Lactulose
(d) Aluminum hydroxide
(e) Metronidazole

38 (a) **True** – Non steroidal anti-inflammatory drugs (NSAIDs) cause salt and water retention, and reduce renal blood flow by inhibition of prostacyclin and prostaglandin E_2 synthesis in patients with renal compromise. This disrupts autoregulation of renal blood flow and GFR thus preventing the normal physiological mechanism which ensures preferential perfusion of the functioning kidney. NSAIDs are less commonly associated with papillary necrosis or interstitial nephritis

(b) **False**

(c) **True** – Radiographic contrast media cause a transient decrease in GFR. The mechanism is unknown

(d) **True** – Angiotensin-converting enzyme (ACE) inhibitors, although often effective in treating heart failure and hypertension in patients with renal disease, can impair renal function. They must be avoided in bilateral renal artery stenosis

(e) **True** – Can cause acute tubular necrosis and renal tubular acidosis

39 (a) **False** – Spironolactone, an aldosterone antagonist, is effective in reducing ascites. Secondary hyperaldosteronism is a feature of hepatic failure

(b) **True** – Chlorpromazine is hepatotoxic and can precipitate coma

(c) **False** – Lactulose is commonly used to reduce ammonia production

(d) **True** – Aluminum hydroxide causes constipation which indirectly increases plasma ammonia

(e) **False** – Metronidazole is commonly used against anaerobic bacteria in severe liver disease but the dose should be decreased

40 Monitoring drug concentrations of the following drugs is recognized as a valuable supplement to clinical monitoring:

(a) Carbimazole
(b) Warfarin
(c) Gentamicin
(d) Lithium
(e) Cyclosporin (ciclosporin)

41 The following are associated with a decreased clearance of theophylline:

(a) Cirrhosis
(b) Heart failure
(c) Gilbert's syndrome
(d) Concurrent phenobarbitone
(e) Smoking

42 In pregnancy:

(a) Most drugs cross the placenta by active transport
(b) Ionized drugs cross the placenta more easily than unionized drugs
(c) Drugs that reduce placental blood flow can reduce birth weight
(d) The fetal blood–brain barrier is not developed until the second half of pregnancy
(e) The human placenta metabolizes endogenous steroids

GENERAL PRINCIPLES

40 (a) **False** – Carbimazole is an anti-thyroid drug. The effective dose is
determined by monitoring blood thyroid function tests.
Carbimazole should be stopped promptly if there is clinical
or laboratory evidence of neutropenia

(b) **False** – Warfarin therapy is monitored by measurement of
prothrombin time (INR)

(c) **True** – Gentamicin "peak" concentrations (30 minutes after dose)
correlate with efficacy, trough concentrations correlate with
toxicity. Aminoglycosides are associated with ototoxicity and
nephrotoxicity

(d) **True** – Insidious increases in serum lithium concentrations can lead
to coma and convulsions

(e) **True** – Not only does cyclosporin show marked interindividual
variability but also compliance is a particular problem in
children. Deterioration in renal function post-transplant may
reflect either graft rejection possibly associated with low
cyclosporin concentrations or toxicity from excessive
concentrations

41 (a) **True**   Theophylline has a narrow therapeutic window and plasma
(b) **True**   concentrations are affected by many factors. High concentra-
(c) **False**   tions are associated with convulsions and arrhythmias. Of
(d) **False**   major concern is the asthmatic on oral theophylline who may
(e) **False**   take additional theophylline because of deteriorating asthma
who is then given intravenous theophylline in casualty.
Phenobarbitone induces CYP_{450} and increases theophylline
clearance; so does smoking.

42 (a) **False**   Most drugs cross the placenta (a cellular membrane) by
(b) **False**   passive diffusion down a concentration gradient. Lipid
(c) **True**   solubility enhances transport across membranes and drugs in
(d) **True**   the unionized state are more lipid soluble. The human
(e) **True**   placenta possesses multiple enzymes.

43 The following drugs are confirmed teratogens in humans:

    (a) Alcohol
    (b) Warfarin
    (c) Isotretinoin
    (d) Paracetamol (acetaminophen)
    (e) Amoxicillin

44 During pregnancy:

    (a) Gastric emptying and small intestinal motility are reduced
    (b) Blood volume increases
    (c) Plasma volume increases
    (d) Predominantly water-soluble drugs will have a larger apparent volume of distribution
    (e) Phenytoin metabolism is inhibited

45 During pregnancy:

    (a) Renal plasma flow increases
    (b) Glomerular filtration rate increases
    (c) Digoxin excretion increases
    (d) Lithium excretion increases
    (e) Gentamicin excretion increases

43 (a) **True** – The risk of having an abnormal baby is about 10% in mothers drinking 30–60 mL ethanol per day rising to 40% in chronic alcoholics

  (b) **True** – Warfarin has been associated with nasal hypoplasia and chondrodysplasia when given in the first trimester and with CNS abnormalites and hemorrhagic complications in later pregnancy. Neonatal hemorrhage is difficult to prevent because of the immature enzymes in fetal liver and low stores of vitamin K

  (c) **True** – Isotretinoin is a teratogen. Effective contraception must be used for at least 1 month before, during, and at least 1 month after oral treatment

  (d) **False** – The minor analgesic of choice in pregnancy

  (e) **False** – Commonly used to treat urinary tract infection in pregnancy

44 (a) **True** – This is of little consequence unless rapid drug action is required. Vomiting associated with pregnancy occasionally makes oral administration impractical

  (b) **True** – Blood volume in pregnancy increases by one-third

  (c) **True** – Plasma volume increases from 2.5 to 4 litres at term and is disproportionate to the expansion in red cell mass so the hematocrit falls

  (d) **True** – Edema, which at least one-third of women experience during pregnancy, may add up to 8 litres to the volume of extracellular water. For water-soluble drugs (which usually have a relatively small volume of distribution) this increases the volume of distribution

  (e) **False** – Metabolism of drugs by the pregnant liver is increased

45 (a) **True**   Excretion of drugs via the kidney increases because renal

  (b) **True**   plasma flow almost doubles and the glomerular filtration

  (c) **True**   rate increases by two-thirds during pregnancy.

  (d) **True**

  (e) **True**

nutritionals	per 100g	per punnet
Energy (kJ)	2110 kJ	779 kJ
Energy (kcal)	503 kcal	186 kcal
Fat	34 g	12 g
of which saturates	12 g	4.4 g
Carbohydrate	29 g	11 g
of which sugars	17 g	6.5 g
Fibre	17 g	6.3 g
Protein	13 g	4.7 g
Salt	0.20 g	0.08 g

ingredients:
dark chocolate buttons (36%) - cocoa mass, dietary fibre (oligofructose), fat-reduced cocoa powder, milk fat, sugar, emulsifier: sunflower lecithin, natural vanilla flavouring (minimum cocoa solids 94.6%)

chewy banana coins (23%)

cocoa dusted almonds (23%) - **almonds**, plain chocolate (cocoa mass, sugar, fat-reduced cocoa powder, emulsifier: **soya** lecithin, natural vanilla flavouring (minimum cocoa solids 70%)), cocoa powder, stabiliser: gum arabic

baked salted peanuts (18%) - blanched **peanuts** (98%), salt (1%), tapioca starch

2 x 37g Best before: 02/01/2021

choccy wonders - pretzel & hazelnut

nutritionals	per 100g	per punnet
Energy (kJ)	2160 kJ	670 kJ
Energy (kcal)	516 kcal	160 kcal
Fat	35 g	11 g
of which saturates	10 g	3.1 g
Carbohydrate	32 g	9.9 g
of which sugars	8.0 g	2.5 g
Fibre	16 g	5.1 g
Protein	13 g	4.1 g
Salt	0.46 g	0.14 g

ingredients:
dark chocolate buttons (34%) - cocoa mass, dietary fibre (oligofructose), fat-reduced cocoa powder, milk fat, sugar, emulsifier: sunflower lecithin, natural vanilla flavouring (minimum cocoa solids 94.6%)

pretzel bites (22%) - **wheat** flour, sunflower oil, poppy seeds, **sesame** seeds, salt, malted **wheat** flour, yeast

roasted **hazelnuts** (21%)

vanilla pumpkin seeds (18%) - pumpkin seeds, sugar, glucose, honey, natural vanilla flavouring

Extra nutrients per 100g: Copper 0.54 mg (54% NRV), Manganese 1.3 mg (66% NRV).

nutritionals	per 100g	per punnet	ingredients
Energy (kJ)	kJ	kJ	
Energy (kcal)	kcal	kcal	
Fat	g	g	
of which saturates	g	g	
Carbohydrate	g	g	
of which sugars	g	g	
Fibre	g	g	
Protein	g	g	
Salt	g	g	

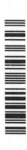

for allergens, including cereals containing gluten, see ingredients in **bold**

All of our food is packed in the same place, so may contain gluten, eggs, peanuts, soya, milk, nuts, celery, mustard, sesame & fish. Watch out for tiny bits of shell or stone in our natural foods – they do sneak past us occasionally.

46 The following are believed safe in pregnancy:

  (a) Penicillins
  (b) Erythromycin
  (c) Fluoroquinolones
  (d) Aminoglycosides
  (e) Ribavirin

47 The following are appropriate in the management of dyspepsia in the second and third trimester:

  (a) Low roughage diet
  (b) Avoidance of fresh fruit and vegetables
  (c) Small, frequent meals
  (d) Misoprostol
  (e) Alginates

48 The following drugs do not cross the placenta in significant amounts:

  (a) Heparin
  (b) Warfarin
  (c) Corticosteroids
  (d) Sodium valproate
  (e) Pethidine

GENERAL PRINCIPLES

46 (a) **True** – Antimicrobials are commonly prescribed in pregnancy
   (b) **True**
   (c) **False** – Minimal experience, animal data discouraging
   (d) **False** – The fetal VIIIth nerve is more sensitive to aminoglycoside toxicity
   (e) **False** – Ribavirin inhibits a wide range of DNA and RNA viruses. It is used by inhalation to treat severe RSV bronchiolitis in children and is used in combination with interferon-α to treat chronic hepatitis C infection. It is a very potent teratogen in animal models. Effective contraception must be ensured for 4 months after treatment in women and 7 months after treatment in men. Condoms must be used if partner of male patient (ribavirin excreted in semen) is pregnant

47 (a) **False** Non-drug treatment – reassurance, small frequent meals and
   (b) **False** advice on posture should be pursued in the first instance.
   (c) **True** Misoprostol, which is an analog of prostaglandin E_1 causes
   (d) **False** abortion.
   (e) **True**

48 (a) **True** – Accumulating evidence suggests this is also true for the low molecular weight heparins (which are often the anticoagulants of choice in pregnancy)
   (b) **False** – Warfarin is a teratogen and is associated with a high incidence of hemorrhagic complications in late pregnancy
   (c) **False**
   (d) **False** – Sodium valproate is an anticonvulsant
   (e) **False** – Pethidine which is commonly used as an analgesic during delivery can cause apnea of the new-born which is reversed with naloxone

49 The use of phenytoin in pregnancy:

(a) Is absolutely contraindicated
(b) Is associated with cleft lip and palate
(c) The "therapeutic" blood concentration of total drug is lower than in the non-pregnant state
(d) Is associated with ataxia if an excessive dose is used
(e) Requires oral vitamin D supplements

50 The following drugs are appropriate for managing hypertension diagnosed in pregnancy in an asthmatic woman:

(a) Bendrofluazide
(b) Atenolol
(c) Labetalol
(d) ACE inhibitors
(e) Methyldopa

51 The following are absolutely contraindicated in pregnancy:

(a) Salbutamol
(b) Corticosteroids
(c) General anesthesia
(d) Quinine
(e) Sucralfate

52 In neonates relative to adults:

(a) Gastric acid is reduced
(b) Fat content (as a percentage of body weight) is low
(c) Plasma albumin concentration is low
(d) The blood-brain barrier is more permeable
(e) The glomerular filtration rate is reduced

GENERAL PRINCIPLES

49 (a) **False** Epilepsy in pregnancy can lead to fetal and maternal
morbidity/mortality through convulsions. Although all anti-
   (b) **True** convulsants are teratogenic the risk of untreated epilepsy is
greater to the mother and fetus than drug-induced
   (c) **True** teratogenicity. To counteract the risk of neural tube defects,
adequate folate supplements are advised. In view of the
   (d) **True** risk of neonatal bleeding associated with carbamazepine,
phenobarbitone and phenytoin; vitamin K is recommended by
   (e) **False** the *BNF* for the mother before delivery (and the neonate).

50 (a) **False** If treatment is initiated during pregnancy it is appropriate to
   (b) **False** use methyldopa which has the longest record of use and
   (c) **False** follow-up in children born to mothers following treatment.
   (d) **False** Beta blockers are contraindicated in asthma. ACE inhibitors
   (e) **True** are teratogens. See *TCP*, Chapter 9, p. 71 and Chapter 27,
pp. 273–275.

51 (a) **False** – Commonly used to treat asthma and occasionally premature
labor
   (b) **False** – Minimal problems when given by inhalation or in short
courses (e.g. to help immature fetal lung) and although cleft
palate and congenital cataract have been attibuted to large
systemic doses of corticosteroids the benefit of treatment
usually outweighs the risk
   (c) **False** – Although there is an increased risk of spontaneous abortion
associated with general anesthesia a causal link is uproven
and in most circumstances failure to operate would have
dramatically increased the risk to mother and fetus
   (d) **False** – Falciparum malaria has a high mortality in pregnancy
   (e) **False** – Sucralfate is not absorbed

52 (a) **True** Neonates are not miniature adults in terms of drug handling
   (b) **True** because of differences in body constitution, drug absorption,
   (c) **True** distribution, metabolism, excretion and sensitivity to adverse
   (d) **True** reactions.
   (e) **True**

53 The following drugs should be avoided during breast feeding:

- (a) Amiodarone
- (b) Carbamazepine
- (c) Ciprofloxacin
- (d) Cyclophosphamide
- (e) Ranitidine

54 The following drugs suppress lactation:

- (a) Anthraquinones (e.g. senna)
- (b) Bromocriptine
- (c) Frusemide (furosemide)
- (d) Salbutamol
- (e) Metronidazole

55 The following properties of a drug encourage their presence in breast milk:

- (a) High lipid solubility
- (b) Unionized state
- (c) Low molecular weight
- (d) Weak base
- (e) Short half-life

53 (a) **True** – Significant concentration in breast milk and there is a theoretical risk from iodine release
   (b) **False** – Minimal concentration in breast milk
   (c) **True** – High concentration in breast milk, animal experiments suggest damage to growing joints
   (d) **True** – Avoid breast feeding
   (e) **False**

54 (a) **False** – But may cause diarrhea in infant
   (b) **True**
   (c) **True**
   (d) **False**
   (e) **False** – But gives milk an unpleasant taste

55 (a) **True**   The total dose of drug in breast milk ingested by the infant is
   (b) **True**   usually too small to cause problems (with some notable
   (c) **True**   exceptions, see Table 1). The infant should be monitored
   (d) **True**   clinically if β-adrenoceptor antagonists are prescribed to the
   (a) **False**   mother. Milk is mildly acid, so weak bases accumulate in it.

Table 1 Some drugs to be avoided during breast feeding

Vitamin A /retinoid analogs	Combined oral contraceptives
Amiodarone	Cyclosporin (ciclosporin)
Aspirin	Cytotoxics
Stimulant laxatives	Ergotamine
Benzodiazepines	Octreotide
Chloramphenicol	Sulfonylureas
Ciprofloxacin	Thiazide diuretics

56 The following are appropriate in the management of acute severe asthma in a 5-year-old child:

(a) Nebulized β_2-agonists
(b) Systemic corticosteroids
(c) Rectal diazepam
(d) Systemic ipratropium
(e) Systemic chlorpheniramine

57 A "normal" man of 75 in comparison with a "normal" man of 35:

(a) Is more likely to be on regular drug therapy
(b) Is more prone to sedation with benzodiazepines
(c) Has a higher endogenous production of creatinine
(d) Has an increased liability to allergic reactions
(e) Usually requires a lower dose of warfarin to achieve anticoagulation

58 The following drugs may precipitate acute retention of urine in the elderly:

(a) Gliclazide
(b) Frusemide (furosemide)
(c) Thioridazine
(d) Amitriptyline
(e) Ampicillin

59 The half-life of the following drugs is increased in the elderly:

(a) Gentamicin
(b) Glibenclamide
(c) Lithium
(d) Dextropropoxyphene
(e) Diazepam

56 (a) **True**
   (b) **True** – A 5-day course of systemic corticosteroids is often sufficient
   (c) **False** – Potentially fatal
   (d) **False**
   (e) **False** – Potentially fatal

57 (a) **True** – See *TCP*, Chapter 11
   (b) **True**
   (c) **False** – One reason why plasma creatinine is a less reliable indicator
              of renal function in the elderly is that endogenous creatinine
              production is reduced
   (d) **True**
   (e) **True** – Probably due to reduced clearance

58 (a) **False** – Gliclazide, a short-acting sulfonylurea, is commonly
              prescribed to elderly diabetics whose blood glucose is
              inadequately controlled by diet alone
   (b) **True**
   (c) **True** – Thioridazine, a phenothiazine which is commonly used to
              treat restlessness and agitated depression in the elderly, has
              anticholinergic effects which may lead to retention of urine
   (d) **True** – Amitriptyline, a sedative tricyclic antidepressent, also has
              anticholinergic effects
   (e) **False**

59 (a) **True** – Related to the decrease in GFR associated with aging
   (b) **True** – Related to the decrease in GFR associated with aging
   (c) **True** – Related to the decrease in GFR associated with aging
   (d) **True** – Related to the decrease in GFR associated with aging
   (e) **True** – Due to the increase in volume of distribution and probably
              also reduced metabolism

60 The following drugs should not be used in those over 75 years old:

(a) Captopril
(b) Finasteride
(c) Streptokinase
(d) Doxycycline
(e) Fluoxetine

61 A woman of 75 is more likely to have the following adverse effects than a woman of 25:

(a) Confusion during treatment with cimetidine
(b) Dystonia during treatment with metoclopramide
(c) Gastrointestinal hemorrhage during treatment with indomethacin
(d) Increased incidence of postural hypotension during phenothiazine therapy
(e) Increased risk of agranulocytosis during clozapine therapy

62 The following are "type A" adverse reactions (i.e. a consequence of the drug's normal pharmacological effect):

(a) Propranolol and fatigue
(b) Chlorpromazine and hepatotoxicity
(c) Naproxen and gastrointestinal hemorrhage
(d) Cyclophosphamide and neutropenia
(e) Diazepam and sedation

63 Stopping treatment with the following drugs may lead to adverse effects due to drug withdrawal:

(a) Prednisolone
(b) Clonidine
(c) Lorazepam
(d) Metoprolol
(e) Ergotamine

60 (a) **False**
   (b) **False** – Finasteride is a specific inhibitor of the enzyme 5α-reductase which metabolizes testosterone into the more potent androgen, dihydrotestosterone
   (c) **False**
   (d) **False** – Doxycycline is a unique tetracycline in that it is not affected by renal function
   (e) **False** – Has fewer anticholinergic effects than most antidepressants

61 (a) **True**
   (b) **False** – Most common in young women
   (c) **True**
   (d) **True** – Impairment of cardiovascular reflexes to erect posture in the elderly is exaggerated by phenothiazines
   (e) **True**

62 (a) **True** – See *TCP*, Chapter 11, pp. 94–95.
   (b) **False**
   (c) **True**
   (d) **True**
   (e) **True**

63 (a) **True** – Prolonged corticosteroid therapy leads to adrenal atrophy and insufficiency. Risks are minimized by the use of steroid cards, using systemic corticosteroids for the minimum period necessary and gradual withdrawal after prolonged therapy. Atrophy may persist for years after stopping corticosteroid therapy and may only be revealed during "stress" (e.g. acute illness/surgery)
   (b) **True** – Rebound hypertension
   (c) **True** – Benzodiazepines cause psychological and physical addiction
   (d) **True**
   (e) **False**

64 The following adverse reactions are associated with the drugs named:

   (a) Oral contraception – gastrointestinal hemorrhage
   (b) Co-amoxiclav – acute liver failure
   (c) Cocaine – stroke
   (d) Thiazide diuretics – impotence
   (e) Prednisolone – osteomalacia

65 The following are examples of type 1 hypersensitivity reaction:

   (a) Penicillin induced anaphylactic shock
   (b) Methyldopa induced Coombs' positive hemolytic anemia
   (c) Hydralazine induced systemic lupus erythematosus
   (d) Amiodarone-induced photosensitivity skin rashes
   (e) Terfenadine-induced ventricular tachycardia

66 The following drugs are associated with erythema multiforme:

   (a) Phenytoin
   (b) Cyclophosphamide
   (c) Salbutamol
   (d) Halothane
   (e) Co-trimoxazole

67 The following drugs are recognized as causing thrombocytopenia:

   (a) Gold salts
   (b) Thiazides
   (c) Heparin
   (d) Aminosalicylates
   (e) Atenolol

68 The following combinations outside the body (e.g. in infusion bag) cause drug inactivation:

   (a) Penicillin and hydrocortisone
   (b) Phenytoin and 5% glucose
   (c) Sodium bicarbonate and calcium chloride
   (d) Erythromycin and 0.9% normal saline
   (e) Heparin and 5% glucose

64 (a) **False** – Oral contraceptive use is associated with thromboembolism
   (b) **True**
   (c) **True** – Also associated with myocardial infarction
   (d) **True**
   (e) **False** – Corticosteroid therapy is associated with osteoporosis. Prolonged use of some anticonvulsants (e.g. phenytoin) is very rarely associated with osteomalacia

65 (a) **True** – Life saving treatment is intramuscular adrenaline
   (b) **False** – A type II reaction
   (c) **False** – A type III reaction
   (d) **False** – A type IV reaction
   (e) **False** – Related to high terfenadine blood concentrations, often as a result of drug interaction through inhibition of CYP3A4

66 (a) **True** – Also associated with acne, coarse facies, hirsutism and toxic epidermal necrolysis
   (b) **False**
   (c) **False**
   (d) **False**
   (e) **True** – Usually due to the sulfamethoxazole but may also be caused by trimethoprim

67 (a) **True** – See *TCP*, Chapter 12, pp. 92–93.
   (b) **True**
   (c) **True**
   (d) **True**
   (e) **False**

68 (a) **True** – Inactivation of penicillin
   (b) **True** – Precipitates
   (c) **True** – Precipitates
   (d) **False**
   (e) **False**

69 Individuals who are "slow acetylators" (i.e. have relatively low activities of hepatic acetyltransferase):

(a) Have prevalence of 5–10% amongst Caucasians in the UK
(b) Are more likely to develop agranulocytosis whilst being treated with clozapine
(c) Are more likely to develop hepatotoxicity after a paracetamol overdose
(d) Are more likely to develop a lupus-like syndrome during hydralazine therapy
(e) Are more likely to develop peripheral neuropathy during isoniazid therapy

70 The following drugs can produce hemolysis in patients with glucose 6-phosphate dehydrogenase (G6PD) deficiency:

(a) Dapsone
(b) Probenecid
(c) Primaquine
(d) Co-trimoxazole
(e) Ciprofloxacin

71 Drug-induced exacerbations of acute porphyria:

(a) Are usually precipitated by enzyme inhibitors (e.g. cimetidine)
(b) Are often precipitated by a single dose of drug
(c) Are accompanied by increased urinary excretion of 5-aminolevulinic acid (ALA) and porphobilinogen
(d) May be precipitated by ethanol
(e) May be precipitated by rifampicin

72 Abnormal pseudocholinesterase:

(a) Is typically inherited as a Mendelian dominant
(b) Results in malignant hyperthermia following exposure to suxamethonium
(c) Causes warfarin resistance
(d) Leads to prolonged paralysis following suxamethonium
(e) Is associated with Alzheimer's disease

69 (a) **False**   Approximately 45% of Caucasians are slow acetylators.
   (b) **False**   Examples of drugs acetylated include: isoniazid, hydralazine
   (c) **False**   phenelzine, dapsone and procainamide. The usual "marker"
   (d) **True**   is the dapsone metabolite ratio in the plasma. The isoniazid
   (e) **True**   peripheral neuropathy can be prevented by prophylactic use
                     of pyridoxine.

70 (a) **True**   The gene for G6PD is located on the X chromosome. G6PD
   (b) **True**   deficiency is more common in people from Mediterranean
   (c) **True**   countries.
   (d) **True**
   (e) **True**

71 (a) **False**   The acute porphyrias are due to hereditary abnormalities in
   (b) **True**   heme biosynthesis and may be precipitated by many drugs
   (c) **True**   (see list in *British National Formulary*), expecially inducers of
   (d) **True** P_{450} enzymes.
   (e) **True**

72 (a) **False**   The usual response to a single intravenous dose of
   (b) **False**   suxamethonium is muscular paralysis for about 6 minutes.
   (c) **False**   The effect is brief due to hydrolysis of suxamethonium by
   (d) **True**   plasma pseudocholinesterase. Approximately 1 in 2500
   (e) **False**   patients have abnormal pseudocholinesterase which may
                     result in prolonged paralysis for 2 hours. Inheritance is
                     Mendelian recessive.

73 Phase 1 studies (i.e. initial studies of drugs in man):

   (a) Always require authorization by the Medicines Control Agency.

   (b) The control group is usually the current drug of choice for the proposed indication

   (c) Always use the oral route of administration

   (d) Only commence after all animal studies have been completed

   (e) Are usually performed in terminal patients

74 The Committee on Safety of Medicines (CSM):

   (a) Is an independent group of clinicians, clinical pharmacologists, toxicologists, pathologists and others who advise the drug licensing authority

   (b) Is financed directly by the UK pharmaceutical industry

   (c) Considers the quality, safety and efficacy of medicinal products

   (d) Considers the investigation, monitoring and response to adverse reactions once a drug has been licensed

   (e) Appoints the local committees on ethical practice

75 The following adverse reactions should be reported to the CSM using the yellow prepaid letter card:

   (a) A transient mild skin rash in a patient taking a new non-steroidal anti-inflammatory drug marked with a '▼' in the *British National Formulary*

   (b) Aggravation of asthma in a known asthmatic with the drug of question "a"

   (c) A convulsion following pertussis vaccination

   (d) Acute anaphylactic shock following intravenous penicillin

   (e) Fatal agranulocytosis associated with clozapine

76 The following licensed drugs are produced by insertion of human genes into bacterial, yeast or mammalion cell lines:

   (a) Human insulin

   (b) Growth hormone

   (c) Factor VIII

   (d) Epoetin

   (e) Interferon

73 (a) **False** – Only requires approval of the MCA (Medicine Control Agency) if patients are the volunteers. This is likely to change under EU directives in 2003

(b) **False** – Placebo is the usual control

(c) **False**

(d) **False**

(e) **False** – Phase 1 studies are usually performed in healthy male adults aged 18–35 years

74 (a) **True**   The CSM in practice is the regulatory review board of the UK

(b) **False**   who advise when certificates to perform clinical trials should

(c) **True**   be issued to pharmaceutical companies and advising,

(d) **True**   following review of all the data from a submission, on the

(e) **False**   granting of a product license which will allow the company to market the drug.

75 (a) **True** – See *TCP*, Chapter 12, pp. 86–87.

(b) **True**

(c) **True**

(d) **True**

(e) **True**

76 (a) **True**   The production of human proteins using recombinant

(b) **True**   DNA/RNA technology not only allows extraction of large

(c) **True**   quantities of natural human proteins but also minimizes

(d) **True**   the risk of blood-borne viral infection such as hepatitis B

(e) **True**   and C and HIV.

CHAPTER TWO

Nervous System

77 The following are causes of insomnia:

(a) Day-time exercise
(b) Left ventricular failure
(c) Caffeine
(d) Depression
(e) Fluoxetine

78 Benzodiazepines:

(a) Potentiate the sedative effects of alcohol
(b) Should only be used as hypnotics for a maximum of 2–4 weeks
(c) Suppress REM sleep
(d) Act by binding to the GABA receptor-chloride channel complex and facilitate the opening of the channel in the presence of GABA
(e) Are anxiolytic

79 Benzodiazepine dependence and withdrawal syndrome:

(a) Benzodiazepine withdrawal symptoms should be treated with buspirone
(b) Fits can occur in the first week after withdrawal
(c) The full withdrawal picture usually appears after an interval of 3–8 weeks
(d) Perceptual distortions are characteristic
(e) Shorter acting benzodiazepines are less likely to cause dependence and should be substituted for long-acting benzodiazepines when withdrawing a patient from benzodiazepines

80 Diazepam:

(a) Has a half-life of less than 20 hours
(b) Can cause anterograde amnesia
(c) Is effective in terminating acute dystonia caused by metoclopramide
(d) Never causes fatal overdose
(e) The major site of metabolism is the liver

77 (a) **False**   It is important to identify the cause of insomnia when it can
   (b) **True**   be treated or avoided. (e.g. pain, dyspnea, nocturia,
   (c) **True**   caffeine and depression). Some individuals need little
   (d) **True**   sleep, shortened sleep time is common in the elderly.
   (e) **True**

78 (a) **True**   Benzodiazepines, whilst being much safer than the
   (b) **True**   barbiturates, still have the problems of dependence,
   (c) **True**   potentiation of alcohol, respiratory depression in
   (d) **True**   overdose and suppressing REM sleep.
   (e) **True**

79 (a) **False** – Buspirone is a non-benzodiazepine anxiolytic drug. It does
                  not have marked hypnotic, anticonvulsant or muscle relaxant
                  properties. It does not alleviate benzodiazepine withdrawal
                  symptoms
   (b) **True**
   (c) **False** – The full withdrawal picture usually appears after an interval
                  of 3–8 days
   (d) **True**
   (e) **False** – It is common practice to substitute shorter-acting with
                  longer-acting benzodiazepines (e.g. temazepam → diazepam)
                  to assist withdrawal

80 (a) **False** – Up to 50 hours, the active desmethyl metabolite has a
                  half-life of 36–200 hours
   (b) **True**
   (c) **True**
   (d) **False** – Usually in combination with alcohol or other drugs
   (e) **True**

81 Temazepam:

(a) Has a shorter half-life than diazepam
(b) Potentiates the effects of alcohol
(c) Causes no "hangover" effect 10 hours post-dosing
(d) Is not addictive
(e) In more potent than lorazepam

82 Chlormethiazole (clomethiazole):

(a) Is not absorbed orally
(b) Has a half-life of approximately 10 hours
(c) In cirrhosis the bioavailability is increased about 10-fold
(d) High doses cause cardiovascular and respiratory depression
(e) Is antagonized by ethanol

83 Promethazine:

(a) Is a GABA agonist
(b) Is available without prescription
(c) Causes dry mouth, constipation and reduced sweating
(d) Liver failure is an absolute contraindication
(e) May cause hallucinations

84 Zopiclone:

(a) Is an ultra short-acting benzodiazepine
(b) Is the hypnotic of choice in a breast-feeding mother
(c) Is a more effective anticonvulsant than clonazepam
(d) Is associated with drug dependence
(e) Can cause confusion

85 The following drugs may mimic some of the common clinical features of schizophrenia:

(a) Levodopa
(b) Salbutamol
(c) LSD
(d) Diamorphine
(e) Methylenedioxymethylamphetamine (MDMA, ecstasy)

81 (a) **True** – 5–6 hours in comparison with 20–50 hours
   (b) **True** – This combination is a cause of fatal overdose as well as disinhibited behavior which may lead to crime or road traffic accidents
   (c) **False** – Patients must be warned not to drive or operate heavy machinery if affected
   (d) **False** – Temazepam is a controlled drug
   (e) **False**

82 (a) **False** – Absorption is rapid with peak plasma levels being obtained at 60 minutes. Chormethiazole undergoes extensive first pass metabolism so oral bioavailability is only approximately 15%
   (b) **False** – The $t\frac{1}{2}$ is 50 minutes. The short $t\frac{1}{2}$ reduces the risk of hangover, ataxia and confusion the next day
   (c) **True** – This results from decreased first pass metabolism
   (d) **True** – Fatalities have occurred because of poorly supervised intravenous infusions. Constant rate infusions lead to accumulation
   (e) **False** – It potentiates the effects of alcohol although it may be used to treat acute alcohol withdrawal

83 (a) **False** – Promethazine is an H_1-antihistamine
   (b) **True**
   (c) **True** – Antimuscarinic effects
   (d) **True** – May cause coma
   (e) **True**

84 (a) **False** Zopiclone is a non-benzodiazepine hypnotic which enhances
   (b) **False** GABA activity. In addition to sedation adverse effects include
   (c) **False** bitter, metallic taste, anorexia, nausea and vomiting, visual
   (d) **True** hallucinations, amnesia, aggression and agitation.
   (e) **True**

85 (a) **True** Occasionally drug-induced hallucinations/psychosis may be
   (b) **False** mistaken for schizophrenia. The hypothesis that chronic
   (c) **True** cannabis use and LSD can cause schizophrenia is
   (d) **False** unproven.
   (e) **True**

86 Blockade of central D_2-receptors:

(a) Parallels the clinical efficacy of the conventional antipsychotic drugs such as chlorpromazine, haloperidol and thioridazine
(b) Induces extra-pyramidal effects
(c) Repeated administration of D_2-antagonists causes an increase in D_2-agonist sensitivity due to an increase in abundance of these receptors
(d) Repeated administration of D_2- antagonists may lead to tardive dyskinesia
(e) Causes a decrease in cardiac output

87 The general principles of management of schizophrenia include:

(a) Treatment should be started in hospital promptly after diagnosis
(b) Chlorpromazine is frequently successful on its own in acute psychotic episodes
(c) Concomitant anticholinergics should be routinely prescribed
(d) Once first-rank symptoms have been relieved most patients can return home on low dose antipsychotic maintenance treatment
(e) Risperidone is an effective alternative to chlorpromazine

88 Chlorpromazine:

(a) Has an antidopaminergic action on the extra-pyramidal system
(b) Has an antidopaminergic action on the mesolimbic system
(c) Has an antidopaminergic action on the chemoreceptor trigger zone
(d) Has moderate antimuscarinic properties
(e) Has α-adrenoreceptor blocking properties

89 Indications for phenothiazines such as chlorpromazine include:

(a) Mania
(b) Angle closure glaucoma
(c) Severe agitation and panic
(d) Aggressive and violent behavior
(e) Malignant neuroleptic syndrome

90 Adverse effects associated with phenothiazines include:

(a) Dry mouth
(b) Blurred vision
(c) Postural hypotension
(d) Impaired temperature control
(e) Jaundice

86 (a) **True**   Prolonged use of D_2-receptor blockers is associated with the
   (b) **True**   onset of tardive dyskinesia which may involve structural
   (c) **True**   brain damage and is often irreversible.
   (d) **True**
   (e) **False**

87 (a) **True**
   (b) **True**
   (c) **False**
   (d) **True**
   (e) **True**   – Risperidone is a recently introduced "atypical" antipsychotic
       agent which appears to be more effective against negative
       symptoms than chlorpromazine and is less likely to cause
       extra-pyramidal adverse effects

88 (a) **True**   – Leading to extra-pyramidal side effects, e.g. parkinsonian
       symptoms, dystonia and akathisia
   (b) **True**   – This may be the site of antipsychotic action
   (c) **True**   – Leading to antiemetic effect
   (d) **True**
   (e) **True**

89 (a) **True**
   (b) **False** – A contraindication
   (c) **True**
   (d) **True**
   (e) **False** – Antipsychotic drugs may cause maligant neuroleptic
       syndrome. This rare syndrome (hyperthermia, varying
       conscious level, rigidity and autonomic dysfunction) may be
       treated with dantrolene or bromocriptine

90 (a) **True**   – Anticholinergic
   (b) **True**   – Anticholinergic
   (c) **True**   – Peripheral α-adrenoceptor blockade
   (d) **True**   – Hypothermia in cold weather, hyperthermia in hot weather
   (e) **True**   – Jaundice occurs in 0.5% of patients taking chlorpromazine. It
       is due to intrahepatic cholestasis and is a hypersensitivity
       phenomenon associated with eosinophilia

91 Contraindications to phenothiazines include:

   (a) Huntington's disease
   (b) Concomitant morphine
   (c) Asthma
   (d) Hepatic impairment
   (e) Bone marrow depression

92 Chlorpromazine:

   (a) Has an oral bioavailability of over 90%
   (b) Has a low volume of distribution (approx. 100 mL/kg)
   (c) Is predominantly eliminated via the kidneys as unchanged chlorpromazine
   (d) Of the chlorpromazine in plasma, 90–95% is bound to plasma proteins
   (e) Usually once daily administration is adequate

93 Flupenthixol (flupentixol):

   (a) Is particularly effective in mania
   (b) May be given once every 2–4 weeks via the intramuscular route for chronic schizophrenia
   (c) Is less sedating than chlorpromazine
   (d) Is more prone than chlorpromazine to produce extra-pyramidal toxicity
   (e) Should not be used in patients with porphyria

94 Clozapine:

   (a) Has weak D_2-blocking activity
   (b) Is effective in up to 60% of patients who have not responded to phenothiazines
   (c) Is effective against negative as well as positive symptoms
   (d) Rarely causes tardive dyskinesia
   (e) Causes blood dyscrasias more commonly than most antipsychotics

NERVOUS SYSTEM

91 (a) **False** – Often used to reduce movement and mental disorders in Huntington's disease
(b) **False**
(c) **False** – Although caution is required in severe respiratory disease
(d) **True**
(e) **True** – May cause blood dyscrasias which can be fatal

92 (a) **False** – Oral bioavailabilty is about 30%
(b) **False** – Volume of distribution is large, approximately 22 L/kg
(c) **False** – Metabolism predominately by hepatic microsomes. Over 70 metabolites have been identified
(d) **True**
(e) **True**

93 (a) **False**   Depot intramuscular preparations such as flupenthixol
(b) **True**   decanoate are valuable in the management of schizophrenia
(c) **True**   for maintenance therapy to ensure compliance which is often
(d) **True**   poor in such patients.
(e) **True**

94 (a) **True**   Clozapine is an "atypical antipsychotic". The term is used
(b) **True**   imprecisely but generally covers those antipsychotic drugs
(c) **True**   whose principal pharmacological effect is not D_2 blockade
(d) **True**   and are rarely associated with extra-pyramidal side effects.
(e) **True**   Neutropenia or agranulocytosis develops in up to 3% of patients taking clozapine for 1 year. Although dystonias and tardive dyskinesias are rare, clozapine is associated with fits in 3–4% of patients and rarely cardiovascular collapse.

95 The following drugs in comparison to chlorpromazine are less likely to cause extrapyramidal side effects:

(a) Haloperidol
(b) Olanzapine
(c) Risperidone
(d) Thioridazine
(e) Fluphenzine

96 The following drugs raise synaptic and/or total brain monoamines:

(a) Reserpine
(b) Amitriptyline
(c) Imipramine
(d) Phenelzine
(e) Amphetamine

97 Tricyclic antidepressants:

(a) Are more effective in endogenous rather than reactive depression
(b) Are particularly effective when the depression is associated with psychomotor and physiological changes
(c) Onset of therapeutic action is approximately 2 weeks after starting therapy
(d) Are effective in the management of panic disorder
(e) Are used for the treatment of nocturnal enuresis in children

98 Antidepressants with sedative properties include:

(a) Amitriptyline
(b) Dothiepin
(c) Citalopram
(d) Paroxetine
(e) Sertraline

95 (a) **False** – Haloperidol is a butyrophenone and has similar effects to chlorpromazine but is more sedating and less likely to cause hypotension

(b) **True** – Olanzapine and risperidone are examples of "atypical antipsychotics". These drugs rarely cause extrapyramidal effects but gastrointestinal disturbances, e.g. nausea, are more common with risperidone, whilst increased appetite and weight is associated with olanzapine

(c) **True**

(d) **True** – Thioridazine a "conventional antipsychotic" causes extra-pyramidal effects less frequently than chlorpromazine but there is a high incidence of antimuscarinic effects. Thioridazine may prolong the QT interval and precipitate life-threatening ventricular arrhythmias

(e) **False**

96 (a) **False**   Reserpine depletes neuronal stores of noradrenaline (NA)
   (b) **True**   and 5-hydroxytryptamine (5HT) and causes depression.
   (c) **True**   Tricyclic drugs of the amitriptyline type raise synaptic stores
   (d) **True**   of NA and 5HT and are antidepressant. Monoamine oxidase
   (e) **True**   inhibitors which increase total brain NA and 5HT are also antidepressant. Amphetamine and cocaine raise synaptic NA and alter mood but are not antidepressant.

97 (a) **True**   See *TCP*, Chapter 19. Although clinical experience is most
   (b) **True**   extensive with the tricyclic antidepressants, the side effect
   (c) **True**   profile of selective serotonin reuptake inhibitors is usually
   (d) **True**   less troublesome and these drugs are safer in overdose.
   (e) **True**

98 (a) **True**   The less sedative tricyclic and related antidepressants include
   (b) **True**   desipramine, imipramine, lofepramine and nortriptyline.
   (c) **False**   Protriptyline is a stimulant. The more sedative drugs are
   (d) **False**   preferred for agitated and anxious patients, whilst the less
   (e) **False**   sedative are preferred in withdrawn patients. Citalopram, paroxetine and sertraline are selective serotonin reuptake inhibitors (SSRIs). SSRIs are less sedating than most tricyclic antidepressants. Insomnia occurs in some patients on SSRIs.

99 The following are consistent with tricyclic antidepressant overdose:

    (a) Dilated pupils
    (b) Hyperreflexia
    (c) Sinus tachycardia
    (d) Widened QRS on the ECG
    (e) Convulsions

100 The following effects are associated with tricyclic antidepressants:

    (a) Hypersalivation
    (b) Constipation
    (c) Aggravation of narrow angle glaucoma
    (d) Dry skin due to loss of sweating
    (e) Fine tremor

101 The following are contraindications to imipramine therapy:

    (a) Asthma
    (b) Epilepsy
    (c) Recent myocardial infarction
    (d) Unpaced heart block
    (e) Porphyria

102 Amitriptyline:

    (a) Is highly lipid soluble
    (b) Is highly protein bound
    (c) Has a low volume of distribution (approx. 100 mL/kg body weight)
    (d) Blocks uptake of monoamines into cerebral and other neurons
    (e) Delays gastric emptying

103 Fluvoxamine:

    (a) Inhibits MAO
    (b) Is a powerful anticholinergic agent
    (c) Is less sedative than trazodone
    (d) Inhibits a CYP_{450} isoenzyme
    (e) During therapy the blood count should be monitored weekly

99 (a) **True**   Tricyclic antidepressant overdoses are commonly fatal.
  (b) **True**   Patients may die from cardiac arryhthmias, convulsions or
  (c) **True**   direct CNS depression leading to respiratory arrest/asphyxia.
  (d) **True**   See *TCP*, Chapter 53.
  (e) **True**

100 (a) **False** – Anticholinergic action leads to dry mouth
  (b) **True** – Anticholinergic action
  (c) **True** – Anticholinergic action
  (d) **True** – Anticholinergic action
  (e) **True** – Sympathomimetic action

101 (a) **False** See *TCP*, Chapter 19, p. 157.
  (b) **True**
  (c) **True**
  (d) **True**
  (e) **True**

102 (a) **True**   Amitriptyline is a sedative tricyclic antidepressant which is
  (b) **True**   usually administered as a single nocte dose.
  (c) **False**
  (d) **True**
  (e) **True**

103 (a) **False** – Fluvoxamine is a selective serotonin (5HT) reuptake
            inhibitor
  (b) **False**
  (c) **True**
  (d) **True** – Fluvoxamine inhibits CYP1A2 and therefore decreases the
            metabolism of theophylline and warfarin. Both these drugs
            have a narrow therapeutic index hence their concomitant
            administration with fluvoxamine should be avoided if
            possible
  (e) **False**

104 Fluoxetine:

(a) Selectively blocks neuronal uptake of noradrenaline
(b) Is more cardiotoxic than imipramine
(c) Is less sedative than amitriptyline
(d) Is associated with nausea and dyspepsia
(e) Has a short elimination half-life of 1–2 hours

105 Phenelzine:

(a) Is a reversible selective inhibitor of MAO-B
(b) Onset of therapeutic effect is usually within 1 week
(c) Is ineffective if used alone in the treatment of depression
(d) Is sometimes effective in reducing hypochondriacal and hysterical symptoms
(e) Is more likely to cause a hypertensive crisis when an indirectly acting sympathomimetic (e.g. ephedrine) is given concurrently rather than a directly acting sympathomimetic (e.g. adrenaline)

106 Moclobemide:

(a) Is a reversible selective inhibitor of MAO-A
(b) Is effective adjunct therapy in Parkinson's disease
(c) Has a longer duration of MAO inhibition compared to phenelzine after stopping therapy
(d) Causes dry mouth in over 50% of patients
(e) Is less likely than phenelzine to cause a food (tyramine) interaction

107 The following foodstuffs/chemicals can cause a hypertensive/hyperthermic reaction during non-selective monamine oxidase inhibitor therapy:

(a) Cheese
(b) Yoghurt
(c) Beer
(d) Marmite™
(e) Grouse

104 (a) **False**   Fluoxetine is a selective serotonin (5HT) reuptake
    (b) **False**   inhibitor. It is safer in overdose and causes fewer
    (c) **True**   antimuscarinic side effects than the tricyclic
    (d) **True**   antidepressants. The most common adverse effects related
    (e) **False**   to selective serotonin reuptake inhibitors are nausea,
                  dyspepsia, diarrhea, dry mouth, headache, insomnia and
                   dizziness. Sweating, erectile dysfunction and delayed
                   orgasm are well recognized associations.

105 (a) **False**   Phenelzine (and isocarboxazid and tranylcypromine) are
    (b) **False**   irreversible non-selective MAO inhibitors.
    (c) **False**
    (d) **True**
    (e) **True**   – Adrenaline is metabolized by catechol-*O*-methyltransferase

106 (a) **True**   – Moclobemide is a reversible, competitive, selective MAO
                  inhibitor
    (b) **False**   – Selegiline, a MAO-B inhibitor, is used in Parkinson's disease
    (c) **False**
    (d) **False**   – No anticholinergic action (cf. tricyclic antidepressants)
    (e) **True**

107 (a) **True**   Patients on MAO inhibitors should be given a treatment
    (b) **True**   card which lists necessary precautions. Interactions with
    (c) **True**   foodstuffs, many proprietary preparations and prescribed
    (d) **True**   drugs may cause a hypertensive crisis. Phenotolamine
    (e) **True**   and/or labetalol are effective treatment for such a reaction.

108 Lithium toxicity can be precipitated by:

(a) Sodium depletion
(b) Thiazide therapy
(c) ACE inhibitors
(d) Non-steroidal anti-inflammatory drugs
(e) Atenolol

109 Therapeutic drug monitoring of plasma concentrations of the following drugs is routinely indicated:

(a) Amitriptyline
(b) Phenelzine
(c) Lofepramine
(d) Lithium
(e) Tryptophan

110 Tricyclic antidepressant therapy should not be started within 14 days of therapy with:

(a) Phenelzine
(b) Isocarboxazid
(c) Tranylcypromine
(d) Moclobemide
(e) St John's wort

111 Parkinsonism is associated with the following drugs/poisons:

(a) Atenolol
(b) Quinine
(c) Phenothiazines
(d) Ethanol
(e) Carbon monoxide

112 Muscarinic antagonists (e.g. benzhexol, benztropine):

(a) Are predominantly used in Parkinsonism caused by antipsychotic drugs
(b) Are least effective in the treatment of tremor
(c) Are ineffective in the management of postencephalitic Parkinsonism
(d) Must not be used with levodopa
(e) May cause confusion in the elderly

108 (a) **True**   Lithium salts have a narrow therapeutic index. Lithium
    (b) **True**   concentrations may rise insidiously and once adverse effects
    (c) **True**   such as tremor, ataxia, dysarthria and nystagmus develop
    (d) **True**   treatment must be stopped whilst the serum lithium (avoid
    (e) **False**   lithium heparin tubes to collect plasma) is measured
                    urgently.

109 (a) **False** See *TCP*, Chapter 8.
    (b) **False**
    (c) **False**
    (d) **True**
    (e) **False** – Tryptophan has been withdrawn from general use because
                    of its association with eosinophilic myalgic syndrome

110 (a) **True** – Irreversible non-selective MAO inhibitor
    (b) **True** – Irreversible non-selective MAO inhibitor
    (c) **True** – Irreversible non-selective MAO inhibitor
    (d) **False** – Reversible selective MAO inhibitor
    (e) **False** – St John's wort is a herbal remedy which is popular for self-
                    treatment of depression. It is a potent CYP_{450} enzyme
                    inducer

111 (a) **False**   The toxic causes of Parkinsonism include phenothiazines,
    (b) **False**   butyrophenones, manganese, carbon monoxide poisoning
    (c) **True**   and MPTP, an illicit "designer drug". Although alcohol
    (d) **False**   withdrawal causes a tremor, alcohol and β-blockers
    (e) **True**   reduce benign essential tremor.

112 (a) **True**   Muscarinic antagonists are effective in the treatment of
    (b) **False**   Parkinsonian tremor and to a lesser extent rigidity. They
    (c) **False**   have minimal effects on bradykinesia. Although more
    (d) **False**   commonly prescribed to counteract antipsychotic-drug
    (e) **True**   induced Parkinsonism they may be used alone in idiopathic
                    Parkinsonism and postencephalitic Parkinsonism if tremor
                    is the predominant symptom.

113 The following enhance central dopaminergic activity:

(a) Inhibition of MAO-B
(b) Bromocriptine
(c) Apomorphine
(d) Haloperidol
(e) Intravenous dopamine

114 Levodopa:

(a) Can enter nerve terminals
(b) Is oxidized by MAO to form dopamine
(c) Is antagonized by bromocriptine
(d) Metabolism is reduced by entacapone
(e) May cause dystonic reactions

115 Levodopa:

(a) Is the amino acid precurser of dopamine
(b) Improves bradykinesia and rigidity more than tremor
(c) Levodopa therapy should be initiated with a loading dose
(d) Levodopa should be taken on an empty stomach
(e) Involuntary movements and psychiatric complications are common unwanted effects

116 Bromocriptine:

(a) Stimulates release of endogenous dopamine
(b) Stimulates postsynaptic D_2 receptors
(c) Is used in conjunction with levodopa-dopa decarboxylase inhibitors
(d) Has an antiemetic action
(e) Inhibits the release of prolactin from the pituitary

117 Selegiline:

(a) Selectively inhibits MAO-B
(b) The most common adverse effect is postural hypotension
(c) Is principally eliminated unchanged in the urine
(d) Cannot be prescribed concurrently with levodopa
(e) Cannot be prescribed concurrently with amantadine

113 (a) **True**   Parkinsonism arises because of deficient dopaminergic
   (b) **True**   transmission. Bromocriptine and apomorphine are
   (c) **True**   dopamine receptor agonists. Acetylcholine is antagonistic
   (d) **False**   to dopamine within the striatum.
   (e) **False**

114 (a) **True**   Levodopa (unlike dopamine) can enter nerve terminals in
   (b) **False**   the basal ganglia where it undergoes decarboxylation to
   (c) **False**   form dopamine.
   (d) **True** – Entacapone is a COMT inhibitor
   (e) **True**

115 (a) **True**   The dose of levodopa is titrated upwards balancing efficacy
   (b) **True**   against adverse effects. Nausea and vomiting are reduced by
   (c) **False**   the addition of a dopa decarboxylase inhibitor and taking
   (d) **False**   the drug after food.
   (e) **True**

116 (a) **False**   Bromocriptine is used as an adjunct with levodopa-dopa
   (b) **True**   decarboxylase combinations in patients with severe
   (c) **True**   motor fluctuations. There is great individual variation
   (d) **False**   in its efficacy. Ropinirole is another dopamine D_2 receptor
   (e) **True**   agonist. In addition to being used as an adjunct to
                levodopa it is often used as monotherapy in younger
                patients to reduce the risk of disabling dyskinesia with
                long-term levodopa therapy.

117 (a) **True**   Selegiline, an MAO-B inhibitor, may slow disease
   (b) **False**   progression in idiopathic Parkinson's disease. It usually
   (c) **False**   allows dose reduction and prolongs the duration of action
   (d) **False**   of levodopa. Oral selegiline is well absorbed (100%) and
   (e) **False**   extensively metabolized in the liver. Rarely hypertension has
                been reported. Amantadine (which stimulates release of
                endogenous dopamine) potentiates its anti-Parkinson
                effects.

118 The following drugs reduce spasticity in patients with upper motor neuron lesions:

   (a) Donepezil
   (b) Metoclopramide
   (c) Diazepam
   (d) Baclofen
   (e) Dantrolene

119 Tardive dyskinesia:

   (a) Occurs in about 15% of patients treated with phenothiazines for over 2 years
   (b) Stopping treatment results in slow improvement in approximately 40% of patients
   (c) Dyskinesia may initially worsen after discontinuing treatment
   (d) Consists of rapid involuntary movements of the limbs
   (e) Is treated with botulinum toxin A

120 In myasthenia gravis:

   (a) Therapy is usually initiated with neostigmine
   (b) Thymectomy may be beneficial
   (c) Corticosteroids and azathioprine reduce circulating T cells
   (d) There is increased sensitivity to atenolol
   (e) Corticosteroids can worsen or improve weakness

121 Severe weakness in a patient with myasthenia gravis may be potentiated by:

   (a) Spontaneous deterioration in the natural history of the disease
   (b) Excessive anticholinesterase drug
   (c) Acute infection
   (d) Aminoglycosides
   (e) Fluoxetine

NERVOUS SYSTEM

118 (a) **False**   Donepezil is used for Alzheimer's disease. Treatment of
    (b) **False**   spasticity is seldom very effective, but physiotherapy or
    (c) **True**   limited surgical release procedures have some place. The
    (d) **True**   drugs used to reduce spasticity have considerable
    (a) **True**   limitations. Diazepam is sedative, baclofen is less sedative
                    at equieffective doses but can cause vertigo, nausea and
                    hypotension. Intrathecal baclofen is currently being
                    evaluated. Dantrolene is less useful for spasticity as it
                    markedly reduces muscle power. It is used in the
                    management of neuroleptic malignant syndrome and
                    malignant hyperthermia.

119 (a) **True**   Tardive dyskinesia is thought to result from the
    (b) **True**   development of "denervation hypersensitivity" in
    (c) **True**   dopaminergic postsynaptic receptors of the nigrostriatal
    (d) **False**   pathway following chronic receptor blockade by
    (e) **False**   neuroleptics. It is therefore due to a relative preponderance
                    of dopaminergic effects. Botulinum toxin A is one of the
                    neurotoxins produced by *Clostridium botulinum* and is used
                    to treat blepharospasm, certain other dystonias and
                    dynamic equinus foot deformities due to spasticity in
                    ambulant pediatric cerebral palsy patients. It blocks the
                    release of acetylcholine at the neuromuscular junction and
                    is given by local intramuscular injection. This is a specialist
                    field!

120 (a) **True**   Myasthenia gravis is a syndrome of increased muscle
    (b) **True**   fatigability and weakness of striated muscle and results
    (c) **True**   from an autoimmune process with antibodies to nicotinic
    (d) **False**   acetylcholine receptors.
    (c) **True**

121 (a) **True**   Clinically the distinction between a deficiency (myasthenic
    (b) **True**   crisis) or an excess (cholinergic crisis) may be difficult and
    (c) **True**   improvement with an injection of the very short-acting
    (d) **True**   anticholinesterase edrophonium is diagnostic of
    (e) **False**   myasthenic crisis. Because of its short duration of action,
                    any deterioration of a cholinergic crisis is unlikely to have
                    serious consequences although facilities for artificial
                    ventilation must be available. NB: cholinesterase inhibitors
                    cause pupillary constriction.

122 The following drugs are effective in partial with or without secondary generalized tonic clonic seizures:

(a) Carbamazepine
(b) Valproate
(c) Phenytoin
(d) Lamotrigine
(e) Ethosuximide

123 Phenytoin is indicated in:

(a) Febrile convulsions
(b) Petit mal absences
(c) Tonic clonic seizures
(d) Partial seizures
(e) Trigeminal neuralgia

124 The following are recognized adverse effects associated with phenytoin therapy:

(a) Ataxia
(b) Dysarthria
(c) Acne
(d) Hyperkalemia
(e) Macrocytic anemia

125 The pharmacokinetics of phenytoin are characterized by:

(a) Wide interindividual variation
(b) Less than 10% systemic bioavailability if taken by mouth with food
(c) Two populations – fast and slow acetylators
(d) The half-life is not affected by dose
(e) Once daily dosing is adequate

126 The ratio of unbound to bound phenytoin is increased by:

(a) Uremia
(b) Pregnancy
(c) Concurrent sodium valproate therapy
(d) Concurrent heparin therapy
(e) Migraine

122 (a) **True** Other drugs (not "first choice") used to prevent such
    (b) **True** seizures include: vigabatrin, phenobarbitone, topiramate,
    (c) **True** tiagabine and clobazam.
    (d) **True**
    (e) **False**

123 (a) **False** See *TCP*, Chapter 21.
    (b) **False**
    (c) **True**
    (d) **True**
    (e) **True**

124 (a) **True** High blood concentrations of phenytoin produce a
    (b) **True** cerebellar syndrome, involuntary movements and sedation.
    (c) **True** Macrocytic anemia which responds to folate is common.
    (d) **False** Rashes, fever, hepatitis, gum hypertrophy, hirsutism and
    (e) **True** lymphadenopathy are all well recognized adverse effects of
                  phenytoin.

125 (a) **True** Age, body weight, sex and in particular, saturable
    (b) **False** metabolism which is under polygenic control, contribute to
    (c) **False** the wide variation in handling of phenytoin.
    (d) **False**
    (e) **True**

126 (a) **True** Unbound, free drug is active. The plasma concentration of
    (b) **True** phenytoin includes both bound and unbound drug. If this
    (c) **True** ratio is altered, the therapeutic range should be adjusted
    (d) **False** accordingly.
    (e) **False**

127 Carbamazepine:

    (a) Inhibits GABA transaminase
    (b) Inhibits its own metabolism
    (c) Is effective in temporal lobe epilepsy
    (d) Inhibits the metabolism of warfarin
    (e) Modified release tablets significantly lessen the incidence of dose-related side effects.

128 The following adverse effects are associated with carbamazepine therapy:

    (a) Trigeminal neuralgia
    (b) Sedation
    (c) Dizziness
    (d) Diplopia
    (e) Hyponatremia

129 The following anticonvulsants are effective in absence/myoclonic seizures:

    (a) Valproate
    (b) Lamotrigine
    (c) Ethosuximide
    (d) Phenytoin
    (e) Clonazepam

130 Sodium valproate:

    (a) Is a dopamine antagonist
    (b) Is indicated in tonic-clonic epilepsy
    (c) The commonest adverse effects are dizziness and sedation
    (d) Rarely causes hepatic necrosis
    (e) Is safe in pregnancy

127 (a) **False** In addition to its effectiveness in all forms of epilepsy
    (b) **False** except absence seizures, carbamazepine is effective in
    (c) **True** trigeminal neuralgia. It induces its own metabolism hence
    (d) **False** the half-life after a single dose is 25–60 hours, but on
    (e) **True** chronic dosing this falls to 10 hours.

128 (a) **False** Carbamazepine commonly causes adverse effects but these
    (b) **True** are seldom severe. They are particularly troublesome early
    (c) **True** in treatment and may resolve without alteration of dose
    (d) **True** which is probably related to the induction of its own
    (e) **True** metabolism, although pharmacodynamic tolerance is also a
factor. Carbamazepine therapy should be initiated at a low
dose and titrated upwards slowly depending on response.
Hyponatremia is caused by stimulation of antidiuretic
hormone secretion.

129 (a) **True** Benzodiazepines are anticonvulsant but are often sedative
    (b) **True** at effective doses and on prolonged use tolerance to their
    (c) **True** antiepileptic properties tends to develop. Clonazepam is
    (d) **False** used intravenously in the treatment of status epilepticus
    (e) **True** and orally as maintenance therapy in a wide variety of
seizure types, in particular, the motor seizures of childhood
including absences and infantile spasms. It has a half-life of
30 hours.

130 (a) **False** Sodium valproate is effective against several forms of
    (b) **True** epilepsy. Adverse effects most commonly involve the
    (c) **False** alimentary system. These include nausea, vomiting and
    (d) **True** abdominal pain (which may be reduced by enteric coated
    (e) **False** tablets). Use in pregnancy is associated with increased
neural tube defects. To reduce the risk of neural tube
defects, folate supplements are advised before and during
pregnancy in women on anti-epileptic drugs.

131 Vigabatrin:

    (a) Is a structural analog of GABA
    (b) Increases the brain concentration of GABA
    (c) Can cause visual field defect
    (d) May cause hallucinations and paranoia
    (e) Is excreted unchanged by the kidney

132 The following anticonvulsants induce the metabolism of estrogen and can lead to unwanted pregnancies in women using oral contraception:

    (a) Carbamazepine
    (b) Phenytoin
    (c) Sodium valproate
    (d) Phenobarbitone
    (e) Lamotrigine

133 An 18-year-old man is admitted to casualty in status epilepticus. There is a history of three previous unexplained blackouts in the last year. The following are appropriate:

    (a) Intravenous diazepam
    (b) Intramuscular phenytoin
    (c) Measurement of blood glucose
    (d) Administration of 24% oxygen
    (e) Once the acute episode is over oral gabapentin should be commenced

131 (a) **True**   Vigabatrin is reserved for the treatment of epilepsy
    (b) **True**   unsatisfactorily controlled by more established drugs. It is
    (c) **True**   associated with visual field defects. Onset of symptoms
    (d) **True**   varies from one month to several years after starting
    (e) **True**   treatment.

Table 2 Choice of drug in various forms of seizure

Form of seizure	First choice	Other drugs
Partial with or without secondary generalized tonic-clonic seizures	Carbamazepine Valproate Phenytoin	Vigabatrin Lamotrigine Phenobarbitone / primidone Clobazam / clonazepam Topiramate Tiagabine
Primary generalized seizures (tonic-clonic)	Valproate	Phenytoin Lamotrigine Clobazam / clonazepam Phenobarbitone / primidone Topiramate
Absence / myoclonic	Valproate Lamotrigine	Ethosuximide Clobazam / clonazepam

132 (a) **True**   Women on long-term enzyme-inducing drugs who are
    (b) **True**   unable to use an alternative reliable method of
    (c) **False**   contraception should use an oral contraceptive containing
    (d) **True**   at least 50 μg ethinylestradiol under expert family planning
    (e) **False**   supervision. Enzyme induction is also the basis of
                    anticonvulsant osteoma lacia (extremely rare) due to
                    reduced serum 25-hydroxycholecalciferol.

133 (a) **True**   Status epilepticus is a medical emergency with a mortality
    (b) **False**   of about 10%. Rapid suppression of seizure activity can
    (c) **True**   usually be achieved with intravenous diazepam (usually
    (d) **False**   10 mg formulated as an emulsion). False teeth should be
    (e) **False**   removed, an airway established and oxygen (60%)
                    administered as soon as possible.

134 **Febrile convulsions:**

(a) Approximately 3% of children have at least one febrile convulsion
(b) A prolonged convulsion can usually be terminated with rectal diazepam
(c) Paracetamol is contraindicated in children who have febrile convulsions
(d) Regular prophylaxis with phenobarbitone reduces the likelihood of adult epilepsy
(e) Children with recurrent febrile convulsions should take prophylactic penicillin

135 **In acute migraine the following are correct:**

(a) Paracetamol or aspirin is usually the treatment of choice
(b) Metoclopramide may be effective due to its dopamine agonist action
(c) Ergotamine may be given by the rectal route
(d) Sumatriptan probably works through its $5HT_{1D}$-agonist properties
(e) Pizotifen is effective when given by intramuscular injection during the acute episode

136 **Sumatriptan:**

(a) Has a greater bioavailability after subcutaneous injection than oral administration
(b) Is contraindicated in patients with ischemic heart disease
(c) Causes a significant, but transient, pressor response
(d) Should not be combined with ergotamine
(e) Metabolism is inhibited by paracetamol

137 **The following are used in the prophylaxis of migraine:**

(a) Sumatriptan
(b) Ergotamine
(c) Pizotifen
(d) Propranolol
(e) Methysergide

134 (a) **True**   Uncomplicated febrile seizures have an excellent prognosis.
(b) **True**   It is usual to reduce fever using paracetamol, removal of
(c) **False**   clothing, tepid sponging and fanning.
(d) **False**
(e) **False**

135 (a) **True**   Oral aspirin or paracetamol is effective in the treatment of
(b) **False**   the headache of acute migraine in nearly 75% of patients.
(c) **True**   During a migraine attack, gastric statis occurs hence the
(d) **True**   popularity of a combination of aspirin or paracetamol with
(e) **False**   metoclopramide (a dopamine antagonist) which enhances
gastric emptying as well as counteracting the nausea
common in migraine. The value of ergotamine is very
limited. There is a risk of peripheral vasospasm.

136 (a) **True**   Sumatriptan is a selective agonist of $5HT_{1D}$-receptors which
(b) **True**   are found predominantly in the cranial circulation.
(c) **True**   Prepacked dosage vials are available for subcutaneous
(d) **True**   self-injection. Sumatriptan is only 14% available after oral
(e) **False**   administration. The half-life is 2 hours. Headache recurs
after a single dose in 30–40% of patients.

137 (a) **False**   Pizotifen is given at night as its principal adverse effect is
(b) **False**   drowsiness. It also increases appetite and causes weight
(c) **True**   gain. Beta-blockers potentiate the peripheral
(d) **True**   vasoconstriction caused by ergotamine and these drugs
(e) **True**   should not be given concurrently. Ergotamine must not be
used for prophylaxis. Methysergide has $5HT_2$-antagonist
activity with partial 5HT-agonist activity. It should only be
used under specialist hospital supervision. Retroperitoneal
fibrosis may lead to renal failure.

138 Halothane:

   (a) Has powerful analgesic properties
   (b) Warning signs of overdosage include bradycardia, hypotension and tachypnea
   (c) Is useful when quiet spontaneous respiration is required
   (d) Increases cerebral blood flow
   (e) Is contraindicated in children

139 Of halothane, enflurane and isoflurane:

   (a) Halothane is most likely to cause hepatic necrosis
   (b) Isoflurane is the least likely to cause cardiac dysrhythmias
   (c) Halothane is used if rapid recovery is important
   (d) Enflurane is the most potent anticonvulsant
   (e) Isoflurane is the agent of choice during neurosurgery

140 Nitrous oxide:

   (a) Has powerful analgesic properties
   (b) Is a powerful muscle relaxant
   (c) After cessation of administration, diffusion hypoxia may occur
   (d) Is contraindicated if pethidine has been administered
   (e) Should not be premixed with oxygen

141 Propofol in comparison to sodium thiopentone:

   (a) Cannot be used for induction of anesthesia
   (b) Has a longer elimination half-life
   (c) Has no active metabolites
   (d) Is less irritant
   (e) Produces a more rapid "clear headed" recovery

142 The following agents are commonly used as premedication for anesthesia:

   (a) Hyoscine
   (b) Temazepam
   (c) Morphine
   (d) Neostigmine
   (e) Ketamine

138 (a) **False**   Halothane is a potent anesthetic but weak analgesic. It has
    (b) **True**   a low therapeutic index. Isoflurane has replaced halothane
    (c) **True**   as the inhalational anesthetic of choice for many
    (d) **True**   indications in the UK.
    (e) **False**

139 (a) **True**   Halothane rarely produces massive hepatic necrosis but
    (b) **True**   much more commonly produces subclinical hepatitis.
    (c) **False**   Enflurane and isoflurane are popular when multiple
    (d) **False**   anesthetics are used and rapid recovery is important.
    (e) **True**   Isoflurane is the least likely to cause dysrhythmias and has
                     the least effect on cerebral blood flow. Sevoflurane is
                     another inhalational agent that has cardiac stability.

140 (a) **True**   Nitrous oxide is commonly combined with volatile
    (b) **False**   anesthetics for its analgesic properties. Premixed nitrous
    (c) **True**   oxide and oxygen mixtures are used in obstetric practice
    (d) **False**   and by ambulance drivers.
    (e) **False**

141 (a) **False**   Sodium thiopentone, an ultra short-acting barbiturate, is
    (b) **False**   used primarily as an induction agent. Propofol is used both
    (c) **True**   for induction, maintenance of anesthesia and sedation on
    (d) **True**   intensive care units.
    (e) **True**

142 (a) **True**   The chief aim of premedication is to allay anxiety in the
    (b) **True**   patient awaiting surgery. Inadequate premedication may
    (c) **True**   lead to the administration of larger doses of anesthetic
    (d) **False**   than would otherwise have been required resulting in
    (e) **False**   delayed recovery. Neostigmine, an anticholinesterase, may
                     be used at the end of a procedure to reverse
                     non-depolarizing muscle relaxants such as tubocurarine.
                     Ketamine is a parenteral anesthetic which has a wide
                     therapeutic index. Although it is a potent analgesic and
                     sedative it can cause vivid unpleasant hallucinations which
                     may recur for months. It increases muscle tone and blood
                     pressure. It is useful in major disasters for rapid, safe
                     anesthesia of trapped casualties to carry out procedures
                     such as amputation.

143 Atracurium:

(a) Is a non-depolarizing muscle relaxant
(b) Has histamine-blocking properties
(c) May be used as a continuous infusion in intensive care to facilitate intermittent positive pressure ventilation
(d) Is metabolized in the liver
(e) Patients with reduced renal function show reduced elimination and prolonged neuromuscular blockade

144 The following would be suitable for postoperative analgesia in a patient with severe chronic obstructive airways disease with CO_2 retention who has had an abdominoperineal resection:

(a) Intramuscular morphine
(b) Epidural block with bupivacaine
(c) Rectal diclofenac
(d) Intramuscular diclofenac
(e) Oral co-proxamol

145 The following are indicated in the management of malignant hyperthermia due to volatile anesthetics or suxamethonium:

(a) Discontinuation of anesthetic
(b) 100% Oxygen
(c) Intravenous dantrolene
(d) Correction of acidosis and hyperkalemia
(e) Cooling

146 Lignocaine (lidocaine), a local anesthetic:

(a) Prevents the rapid inflow of sodium ions which is the ionic basis of the action potential
(b) Causes vasoconstriction
(c) Is not absorbed from the urethra
(d) Can be combined with adrenaline for digital "ring" blocks
(e) Has a shorter duration of action than bupivacaine

143 (a) **True**
(b) **False**
(c) **True**
(d) **False**
(e) **False**

Atracurium has a rapid onset of action. It occasionally causes histamine release leading to flushing of the face and chest, hypotension and rarely bronchospasm. Continuous infusion is popular in intensive care. It is inactivated spontaneously in the plasma which is a valuable property in hepatic and renal failure.

144 (a) **False**
(b) **True**
(c) **False**
(d) **True**
(e) **False**

Opioids may cause fatal respiratory depression. Even epidural opioids can depress respiration and in this situation epidural "local" anesthesia and intramuscular non-steroidal anti-inflammatory drugs are preferred.

145 (a) **True**
(b) **True**
(c) **True**
(d) **True**
(e) **True**

Malignant hyperthermia is a rare but potentially lethal complication of anesthesia. It consists of a rapid increase in body temperature accompanied by tachycardia and generalized muscle spasm. Severe acidosis and hyperkalemia occur. Dantrolene reverses the muscle spasm.

146 (a) **True**
(b) **False**
(c) **False**
(d) **False**
(e) **True**

Small unmyelinated fibers are depressed first hence the order of loss of function is pain, temperature, touch, proprioception and motor function. Lignocaine does not affect vascular smooth muscle but is available with adrenaline, a vasoconstrictor which prolongs its local effect. This combination may cause vasospasm and severe digital ischemia if used for a "ring" block hence the combination is contraindicated in this situation. Bupivacaine is a long-acting local anesthetic which is often used for peripheral nerve, plexus, epidural and spinal anesthesia. Toxicity includes cardiac arrhythmias.

147 The following drugs are correctly paired with their putative site(s) of action:

(a) Non-steroidal anti-inflammatory drugs – at the site of injury, by interfering with the chemical mediators involved in nociception
(b) Paracetamol – peripheral inhibition of cyclo-oxygenase
(c) Lignocaine – block of transmission in peripheral nerves
(d) Opioids – modification of transmission at the dorsal horn
(e) Opioids – interference with central appreciation of pain and inhibition of emotional concomitants

148 Aspirin:

(a) Inhibits cyclo-oxygenase irreversibly
(b) Produces its major analgesic and anti-inflammatory effects by inhibition of prostaglandin E_2 and prostacyclin biosynthesis
(c) Impairs color vision
(d) Acts on the hypothalamus to reduce body temperature
(e) Chronic use is associated with iron deficiency anemia

149 Adverse effects associated with salicylates include:

(a) Claudication
(b) Bronchoconstriction
(c) Systemic lupus erythematosus
(d) Hepatitis
(e) Reye's syndrome

150 Ibuprofen:

(a) Is a reversible cyclo-oxygenase inhibitor
(b) Has analgesic properties
(c) Has antipyretic properties
(d) Has anti-inflammatory properties
(e) Can cause renal impairment

151 Nefopam:

(a) Is associated with gastrointestinal hemorrhage
(b) Causes meiosis
(c) Causes more respiratory depression than morphine
(d) Potentiates the arrhythmogenic effect of halothane anesthesia
(e) Is contraindicated in epilepsy

147 (a) **True**   Paracetamol probably produces its analgesic effect by
   (b) **False**   central inhibition of cyclo-oxygenase. It is antipyretic but
   (c) **True**   not anti-inflammatory.
   (d) **True**
   (e) **True**

148 (a) **True**   Gastric irritation is reduced by taking aspirin after food.
   (b) **True**
   (c) **False**
   (d) **True**
   (e) **True**

149 (a) **False**   The commonest adverse effect associated with salicylates is
   (b) **True**   dyspepsia. Chronic blood loss from the stomach may be
   (c) **False**   asymptomatic. Salicylism which is associated with high
   (d) **True**   blood concentrations consists of tinnitus, deafness, nausea,
   (e) **True**   vomiting and occasionally abdominal pain and flushing.

150 (a) **True**   Ibuprofen is a non-steroidal anti-inflammatory drug which
   (b) **True**   is available without prescription. The side effects are those
   (c) **True**   of all the NSAIDs of which gastrointestinal irritation is the
   (d) **True**   most common. Selective inhibitors of cyclo-oxygenase 2
   (e) **True**   (COX 2), e.g. rofecoxib and celecoxib, may improve
               gastrointestinal tolerance.

151 (a) **False**   Nefopam is chemically and pharmacologically unrelated to
   (b) **False**   opioids and NSAIDs. It is used for moderately severe pain.
   (c) **False**   It can cause fatal hypertension if prescribed during or
   (d) **True**   within 2 weeks of cessation of non-selective MAO inhibitor
   (e) **True**   treatment.

152 Co-proxamol contains:

(a) Aspirin
(b) Paracetamol
(c) Dextropropoxyphene
(d) Caffeine
(e) Promethazine

153 Morphine:

(a) Acts as an agonist at opioid receptors (especially μ) in the brain and spinal cord
(b) Causes pupillary constriction by stimulation of the Edinger–Westphal nucleus in the mid-brain
(c) Acts as an antihistamine
(d) Is subject to presystemic metabolism
(e) Stimulates the chemoreceptor trigger zone

154 The following are particularly sensitive to the pharmacological actions of morphine:

(a) Young children
(b) The elderly
(c) Patients with hepatic failure
(d) Patients with renal failure
(e) Patients with hyperthyroidism

155 Morphine causes:

(a) Diarrhea
(b) Increased intrabiliary pressure
(c) Histamine release
(d) Reduced sensitivity of the respiratory center to carbon dioxide
(e) Vasoconstriction

156 Diamorphine:

(a) Is metabolized to morphine and 6-acetylmorphine
(b) Has a half-life after intravenous injection of approximately 3 minutes
(c) Has a less rapid clinical effect than morphine
(d) Is contraindicated in left ventricular failure
(e) Is antagonized by naloxone

152 (a) **False** Co-proxamol, a compound analgesic of
    (b) **True**   dextropropoxyphene and paracetamol, is widely prescribed.
    (c) **True**   It is dangerous in overdose (see *TCP*, Chapter 53). When
    (d) **False** taking a drug history one must be aware that many
    (e) **False** over-the-counter remedies contain a surprising mixture of
                   pharmacologically active agents, although often in almost
                   "homeopathic" quantities.

153 (a) **True**   The most important use of morphine is pain relief. It is of
    (b) **True**   particular value in palliative care. The use of oral modified
    (c) **False** release preparations allows twice daily dosing whereas if the
    (d) **True**   standard solution is used it needs to be given every 4 hours.
    (e) **True**

154 (a) **True**   Patients with decreased respiratory reserve and myxedema
    (b) **True**   are also more sensitive.
    (c) **True**
    (d) **True**
    (e) **False**

155 (a) **False** Morphine increases smooth muscle tone throughout the
    (b) **True**   gastrointestinal tract and in addition reduces peristalsis
    (c) **True**   through an action on the receptors in the ganglion plexus
    (d) **True**   in the gut wall which results in constipation.
    (e) **False**

156 (a) **True**   Diamorphine is diacetylmorphine. Its actions are similar to
    (b) **True**   those of morphine but is more potent as an analgesic when
    (c) **False** given by injection. It is more soluble than morphine.
    (d) **False** Diamorphine and 6-acetylmorphine enter the brain more
    (e) **True**   rapidly than morphine.

157 Pethidine:

(a) Is more potent than morphine
(b) Does not cause respiratory depression
(c) Always causes pupillary constriction at analgesic doses
(d) Suppresses cough at analgesic doses
(e) Reduces the activity of the pregnant term uterus

158 Codeine:

(a) Is a metabolite of morphine
(b) Has a plasma half-life of approximately 12 hours
(c) Is not antagonized by naloxone
(d) Is used as a cough suppressant
(e) Causes constipation

159 Buprenorphine:

(a) Is a partial agonist on opioid receptors
(b) Occupies a much larger fraction of opioid receptors to produce its analgesic effect than does morphine
(c) Should only be used to treat acute pain
(d) Is subject to prescription requirements under the Misuse of Drugs Act
(e) May be administered sublingually

160 Naloxone:

(a) Binds to opioid μ receptors
(b) Acts as a partial opioid agonist
(c) Has little effect on a healthy person who has not taken opioid drugs
(d) Has an elimination half-life of approximately 12 hours
(e) Is contraindicated in young children

157 (a) **False**   Pethidine causes similar respiratory depression and
    (b) **False**   vomiting to morphine, but does not release histamine or
    (c) **False**   suppress cough and only uncommonly produces pupillary
    (d) **False**   constriction to the same extent as morphine.
    (e) **False**

158 (a) **False**   Morphine is a metabolite of codeine. Codeine is used as an
    (b) **False**   analgesic, cough suppressant and antidiarrheal agent. The
    (c) **False**   plasma half-life is 3–4 hours. It is metabolized by CYP2D6.
    (d) **True**   It is less effective in patients deficient in CYP2D6.
    (e) **True**

159 (a) **True**   In common with other partial agonists buprenorphine
    (b) **True**   occupies a much larger fraction of the receptors to produce
    (c) **False**   its analgesic effect than does a full agonist. Consequently it
    (d) **True**   can precipitate pain and cause withdrawal symptoms in
    (e) **True**   patients who have received other opioids and relatively
                     much larger doses of naloxone are required to displace it
                     from receptors in overdosage compared to a full agonist.

160 (a) **True**   Naxolone is a pure competitive antagonist. It has a half-life
    (b) **False**   of 1 hour which is less than many opioids.
    (c) **True**
    (d) **False**
    (e) **False**

CHAPTER THREE

Musculoskeletal System

161 Ibuprofen:

(a) Inhibits the enzymes cyclo-oxygenase 1 and 2 irreversibly
(b) Inhibits leukotriene biosynthesis
(c) Is a more potent anti-inflammatory agent than indomethacin
(d) May exacerbate or precipitate asthma
(e) Reduces lithium clearance

162 Rofecoxib:

(a) Is a phospholipase A_2 inhibitor
(b) Is a prodrug
(c) Is an effective antiplatelet agent
(d) Is contraindicated in renal failure
(e) Causes gastric erosions less frequently than an equianalgesic dose of ibuprofen

163 The following drugs inhibit both cyclo-oxygenase-1 and 2 (COX 1 and 2):

(a) Diclofenac
(b) Sodium aurothiomalate
(c) Penicillamine
(d) Sulindac
(e) Hydroxychloroquine

164 Gold salts when used in the treatment of progressive rheumatoid arthritis:

(a) Are usually administered daily by intravenous injection
(b) If effective, benefit should be observed after the first week of treatment
(c) Produce objective improvement in 75% of patients
(d) Can cause skin rashes which can necessitate treatment cessation
(e) If they cause stomatitis this may be due to neutropenia

161 (a) **False**   All NSAIDs inhibit cyclo-oxygenase reversibly except aspirin.
    (b) **False**   All NSAIDs have analgesic and anti-inflammatory properties.
    (c) **False**   Inhibition of prostaglandin E_2 biosynthesis is associated
    (d) **True**   with increased leukotriene B_4 biosynthesis.
    (e) **True**

162 (a) **False** – Rofecoxib is a selective COX 2 inhibitor
    (b) **False** – It is the parent compound that is active
    (c) **False** – COX 2 is not expressed in platelets.
    (d) **True** – COX 2 inhibitors can decrease GFR
    (e) **True**

163 (a) **True**   Several drugs are not analgesic and do not inhibit cyclo-
    (b) **False**   oxygenase 1 or 2 but do suppress the inflammatory process
    (c) **False**   in rheumatoid arthritis, e.g. sodium aurothiomalate,
    (d) **True**   penicillamine and hydroxychloroquine. They are often
    (e) **False**   referred to as disease modifying drugs (DMARDS).
                Methotrexate is an immunosuppressant used as a DMARD
                in rheumatoid arthritis. They only have a part to play in
                patients with progressive disease.

164 (a) **False**   Gold (as sodium aurothiomalate) is usually administered as
    (b) **False**   weekly intramuscular injections or by mouth daily. Benefit
    (c) **True**   is not anticipated for at least 6 weeks. Blood dyscrasias and
    (d) **True**   glomerular injury (nephrotic syndrome) occur and
    (e) **True**   monitoring of blood counts and urine is performed
                monthly. Rashes may progress to exfoliation.

165 Penicillamine is used in the management of:

(a) Rheumatoid arthritis
(b) Systemic lupus erythematosus (SLE)
(c) Wilson's disease
(d) Cystinuria
(e) Lead poisoning

166 Adverse effects associated with penicillamine include:

(a) Thrombocytopenia
(b) Leukopenia
(c) Immune complex glomerulonephritis
(d) Loss of taste
(e) Myasthenia gravis

167 Etanercept:

(a) Is a humanized monoclonal antibody against TNF-α
(b) Can cause life-threatening hypersensitivity reactions
(c) Has a half-life of 5–13 days
(d) Can cause pancytopenia
(e) Is rarely associated with a demyelinating syndrome

168 The following are likely to be effective in the treatment of an acute episode of gout:

(a) Indomethacin
(b) Naproxen
(c) Alendronate
(d) Probenecid
(e) Colchicine

169 The following may cause hyperuricemia:

(a) Sulfinpyrazone
(b) Cytosine arabinoside when treating acute leukemia
(c) Bendrofluazide
(d) Low dose aspirin
(e) Bezafibrate

165 (a) **True**   Penicillamine, a breakdown product of penicillin, is given
    (b) **False**   by mouth. In rheumatoid arthritis clinical improvement is
    (c) **True**   anticipated only after 6–12 weeks. It is contraindicated in
    (d) **True**   SLE. Apart from its immunosuppressive action, it also
    (e) **True**   chelates certain heavy metals (Cu, Pb, etc.).

166 (a) **True**   The toxicity of penicillamine is such that it should only be
    (b) **True**   used by clinicians with experience of the drug and with
    (c) **True**   meticulous patient monitoring.
    (d) **True**
    (e) **True**

167 (a) **False** – Etanercept is a recombinant protein that has two soluble
                    TNF receptors joined to an Fc fragment, this is in contrast
                    to infliximab a humanized murine monoclonal against
                    TNF-α used in Crohn's disease. Both are licensed for the
                    treatment of adult rheumatoid arthritis.
    (b) **True** – Like all proteins it can cause hypersensitivity reactions
    (c) **True** – It has a long half-life in plasma and is administered every 2
                    weeks
    (d) **True** – It can cause bone marrow suppression (all lineages) and
                    sepsis
    (e) **True** – Rarely demyelinating syndromes like MS have been
                    reported with its use

168 (a) **True**   Acute gout is treated by anti-inflammatory analgesic
    (b) **True**   agents. Colchicine is an alternative in those unable to
    (c) **False**   tolerate NSAIDs but commonly causes diarrhea.
    (d) **False**   Alendronate is a bisphosphonate used in the management
    (e) **True**   of Paget's disease. Bisphosphonates are also used to treat
                    hypercalcemia of pregnancy. They may be used in the
                    prevention of postmenopausal osteoporosis.

169 (a) **False**   Uric acid is the end product of purine metabolism in
    (b) **True**   humans, and gives rise to problems because of its limited
    (c) **True**   solubility. Cytosine arabinoiside causes massive cell death
    (d) **True**   and increased uric acid production. Diuretics, low dose
    (e) **False**   salicylates and pyrazinamide inhibit tubular excretion of
                    uric acid. Pyrazinamide is used in the treatment of
                    tuberculosis in combination with other drugs.

170 Allopurinol:

(a) Inhibits xanthine oxidase
(b) May precipitate acute gout
(c) Is contraindicated in renal failure
(d) Should not be prescribed with an NSAID
(e) Blocks the inactivation of warfarin

171 In a patient with osteoarthritis:

(a) Physical exercise and weight loss can be helpful
(b) NSAIDs are contraindicated
(c) Gold therapy reverses the pathophysiology of the disease
(d) Symptoms are exacerbated by bisphosphonates, e.g. alendronate
(e) Raloxifene may slow disease progression

172 Indomethacin causes the following adverse effects:

(a) Biochemical hepatitis
(b) Spuriously increases serum creatinine
(c) Hypokalemia
(d) Exacerbates cardiac failure
(e) Antagonizes the antihypertensive effects of ACE inhibitors

170 (a) **True**   Allopurinol is used as long-term medication to treat
    (b) **True**   patients with recurrent gout. By inhibiting xanthine
    (c) **False**   oxidase it decreases uric acid production. It potentiates
    (d) **False**   azathioprine by blocking inactivation of its active
    (e) **False**   metabolite 6-mercaptopurine.

171 (a) **True**
    (b) **False** – NSAIDs are probably one of the most widely used
                    treatments although paracetamol, because of its superior
                    tolerance in the elderly, should be tried first.
    (c) **False**
    (d) **False**
    (e) **False** – Raloxifene is used in the treatment and prevention of
                    postmenopausal osteoporosis

172 (a) **True** – Can cause a transaminitis
    (b) **False** – Reduces GFR and truly causes an increase in serum
                    creatinine by diminishing vasodilatatory prostaglandins in
                    renal bed
    (c) **False** – Reduces renal potassium excretion thus leads to
                    hyperkalemia
    (d) **True** – Reduces Na excretion leading to increased fluid retention
                    and fluid overload
    (e) **True**

CHAPTER FOUR

Cardiovascular System

173 The following are modifiable risk factors for the genesis of atheromatous plaque:

(a) Smoking
(b) Obesity
(c) Dyslipidemia
(d) Glucose intolerance
(e) Hypertension

174 Cholestyramine:

(a) Causes a fall in plasma cholesterol
(b) Increases fecal excretion of bile acids
(c) Reduces absorption of folic acid
(d) Causes diarrhea in diabetic autonomic neuropathy
(e) Reduces pruritus in incomplete biliary obstruction

175 Bezafibrate:

(a) Lowers plasma triglyceride
(b) Is ineffective postcholecystectomy
(c) Inhibits lipoprotein lipase
(d) Is indicated in alcohol-induced hyperlipidemia
(e) Potentiates the effects of warfarin

176 Simvastatin, an HMGCoA reductase inhibitor:

(a) Lowers low density lipoprotein (LDL) cholesterol
(b) Is particularly useful in heterozygous familial hypercholesterolemia
(c) Acts locally on HMGCoA reductase in the intestine
(d) Is associated with myositis/myopathy
(e) Is ineffective if prescribed with a bile acid binding resin

173 (a) **True**   Atheroma is the commonest cause of ischemic heart
    (b) **True**   disease, stroke and peripheral vascular disease.
    (c) **True**
    (d) **True**
    (e) **True**

174 (a) **True**   The anion exchange resins cholestyramine and colestipol
    (b) **True**   are not absorbed into the systemic circulation and bind bile
    (c) **False**   acids in the gut lumen inhibiting reabsorption of bile salts
    (d) **False**   and cholesterol. Cholestyramine causes malabsorption of
    (e) **True**   fat soluble vitamins, and is used to treat pruritus in
                     patients with incomplete biliary obstruction. Side effects
                     include flatulence, constipation and nausea.

175 (a) **True**   The fibrates stimulate lipoprotein lipase and reduce plasma
    (b) **False**   triglyceride. They also tend to reduce LDL cholestrol and to
    (c) **False**   raise HDL cholesterol. They can cause myositis which is
    (d) **False**   more common in alcoholics, patients with impaired renal
    (e) **True**   function and in patients on concurrent HMGCoA reductase
                     inhibitors. Other adverse effects include nausea and
                     abdominal discomfort.

176 (a) **True**   HMGCoA reductase is the rate limiting step in cholesterol
    (b) **True**   biosynthesis from acetate. HMGCoA reductase inhibitors
    (c) **False**   are ineffective in rare patients with homozygous familial
    (d) **True**   hypercholesterolemia as they cannot make LDL receptors.
    (e) **False**

177 The following can cause hypertension:

  (a) Corticosteroid therapy
  (b) Oral contraception
  (c) Alcohol withdrawal
  (d) Opioid withdrawal
  (e) Ergotamine

178 Thiazide diuretics when used in the management of uncomplicated essential hypertension:

  (a) Reduce the risk of stroke
  (b) Are natriuretic
  (c) Potassium supplements are usually required
  (d) Reduce plasma renin
  (e) Are associated with impotence

179 Thiazide diuretics are associated with:

  (a) Purpura
  (b) Hyperuricemia
  (c) Hyperglycemia
  (d) Hypercalcemia
  (e) Hypercholesterolemia

180 Beta-adrenoceptor antagonists:

  (a) Reduce the risk of stroke in hypertension
  (b) Reduce the risk of myocardial infarction in hypertension
  (c) Improve performance of sprinters
  (d) The antihypertensive effect is antagonized by NSAIDs
  (e) May be effectively combined with thiazide diuretics in reducing a raised blood pressure

181 The following drugs when used as monotherapy in the management of hypertension are likely to be less effective in Afro-Caribbeans than in Caucasians:

  (a) Atenolol
  (b) Enalapril
  (c) Bendrofluazide
  (d) Amlodipine
  (e) Doxazosin

177 (a) **True** Although hypertension is usually "essential" (i.e. idiopathic)
    (b) **True** the possibility of secondary hypertension must always be
    (c) **True** considered. Equally important is the confirmation or
    (d) **True** rejection of persistent hypertension by repeated measures
    (e) **True** (blood pressure is very variable) and the identification of
              other treatable risk factors such as diabetes, smoking,
              hypercholesterolemia and obesity.

178 (a) **True** Thiazide diuretics (e.g. bendrofluazide, hydrochlorthiazide)
    (b) **True** remain the logical first choice for treating patients with
    (c) **False** mild hypertension unless contraindicated by some
    (d) **False** co-existent disease and are also valuable in patients with
    (e) **True** more severe hypertension in combination with other
              therapy.

179 (a) **True** Thiazide diuretics are generally well tolerated. Treatment
    (b) **True** should be initated with a low dose (e.g. 2.5 mg bendro-
    (c) **True** fluazide). Higher doses increase the incidence of adverse
    (d) **True** effects relatively more than efficacy. Non-metabolic adverse
    (e) **True** effects include impotence, rashes and thrombocytopenia.

180 (a) **True** The relatively cardioselective β-adrenoreceptor
    (b) **True** antagonists, atenolol and metoprolol, are widely used to
    (c) **False** treat hypertension in the UK. They are particularly valuable
    (d) **True** in patients with angina or who have survived a myocardial
    (e) **True** infarction. Atenolol is a polar drug and undergoes renal
              elimination whilst metoprolol is non-polar and is
              metabolized by CYP_{450} 2D6.

181 (a) **True** Afro-Caribbean patients are less likely to have high
    (b) **True** circulating renin levels hence β-blockers and ACE
    (c) **False** inhibitors are less likely to be effective. This difference is
    (d) **False** statistical and based on large populations and both ACE
    (e) **False** inhibitors and β-blockers can be effective in Afro-Caribbean
              patients but a thiazide is usually the anti-hypertensive of
              first choice.

182 Beta-adrenoceptor antagonists are contraindicated in:

(a) Asthma
(b) Thyrotoxicosis
(c) Second degree heart block
(d) Dissecting thoracic aneurysm
(e) Migraine

183 Captopril, an angiotensin-converting enzyme (ACE) inhibitor:

(a) Reduces concentrations of angiotensin II
(b) Increases concentrations of bradykinin
(c) Increases noradrenaline release from sympathetic nerve terminals
(d) Increases aldosterone secretion
(e) Blocks angiotensin II receptors

184 Captopril is contraindicated in:

(a) Left ventricular failure
(b) Asthma
(c) Bilateral renal artery stenosis
(d) Pregnancy
(e) Diabetic nephropathy

185 Nifedipine, a dihydropyridine calcium channel blocker:

(a) Dilates veins more than arteries
(b) Can be combined with β-blockers in the management of hypertension
(c) Increases plasma calcium concentration
(d) Is contraindicated in diabetes mellitus
(e) Raises the plasma concentration of cholesterol

186 Nifedipine in comparison to verapamil is more likely to:

(a) Worsen angina
(b) Cause ankle swelling unresponsive to diuretics
(c) Have negative inotropic effects
(d) Cause flushing and headache
(e) Cause constipation

182 (a) **True**   In addition to asthma and heart block, β-blockers
    (b) **False**   aggravate peripheral vascular disease and vasospasm and
    (c) **True**   mask the symptoms of hypoglycemia. In some individuals
    (d) **False**   they cause fatigue and hallucinations. They reduce the
    (e) **False**   somatic symptoms of anxiety.

183 (a) **True**   ACE inhibitors inhibit the conversion of inactive
    (b) **True**   angiotensin I to active angiotensin II, a powerful
    (c) **False**   vasoconstrictor, and also inhibit the breakdown of the
    (d) **False**   vasodilator peptides such as bradykinin. This latter effect
    (e) **False**   may cause cough. This may be avoided by using an
          angiotensin II blocker, e.g. losartan, which does not
          potentiate bradykinin.

184 (a) **False**   Plasma creatinine and potassium should be monitored
    (b) **False**   before and during the early weeks of therapy with ACE
    (c) **True**   inhibitors and the possibilty of bilateral renal artery
    (d) **True**   stenosis (one of the few correctable causes of hypertension)
    (e) **False**   considered if there is a marked rise in creatinine.
          Glomerular filtration in these patients is dependent on
          angiotensin-II mediated efferent arteriolar vasoconstriction.
          ACE inhibitors are of particular value in treating diabetic
          hypertensive patients as they significantly slow down the
          progressive renal impairment typical in these patients.

185 (a) **False**   Nifedipine is used in the management of Raynaud's
    (b) **True**   syndrome, hypertension and angina. Modified release
    (c) **False**   tablets are preferred. Amlodipine is a once daily calcium
    (d) **False**   channel blocker with similar properties.
    (e) **False**

186 (a) **True**   Nifedipine, unlike verapamil, has no effect on the
    (b) **True**   conducting system of the heart. In the occasional patient it
    (c) **False**   can worsen angina due to a reflex tachycardia whilst
    (d) **True**   verapamil causes a bradycardia. Both drugs are effective
    (e) **False**   arterial dilators. Verapamil is a much more potent negative
          inotrope.

187 Doxazosin:

(a) Is a selective reversible $\alpha_1$blocker
(b) Should always be prescribed with a β-blocker to prevent reflex tachycardia
(c) Is associated with first dose hypotension
(d) Reduces plasma LDL/HDL cholesterol ratio
(e) Can cause urinary incontinence in women with pre-existing pelvic pathology

188 Sodium nitroprusside:

(a) Is administered by intravenous infusion
(b) Prolonged administration can lead to cyanide poisoning
(c) Has a half-life of about 1 week
(d) Reduces cardiac "pre-load"
(e) Reduces cardiac "afterload"

189 Methyldopa:

(a) Causes central $\alpha_2$agonist effects
(b) Causes drowsiness and fatigue
(c) Pyrexia is an adverse effect
(d) Is associated with Coombs positive hemolytic anemia
(e) A single missed dose can cause profound rebound hypertension

190 The following hypotensive combinations are rational when a single drug has not been effective in treating essential hypertension:

(a) Thiazide and atenolol
(b) Thiazide and captopril in an asthmatic
(c) Amiloride and captopril in an asthmatic who has gout
(d) Nifedipine and verapamil in a man who has had thiazide-induced impotence, 2nd degree heart block and captopril-induced rash
(e) Enalapril and doxazosin in a man with prostatism

191 The following drug effects have been correctly paired with the named drug:

(a) Hydralazine – drug-induced SLE
(b) Minoxidil – hirsutism
(c) Captopril – first dose hypotension
(d) Atenolol – tremor
(e) Clonidine – bronchospasm

CARDIOVASCULAR SYSTEM

187 (a) **True**　Non-specific α-blockers such as phenoxybenzamine
    (b) **False**　cause profound postural hypotension and reflex
    (c) **True**　tachycardia. Doxazosin does not block presynaptic
    (d) **True**　α_2-receptors that are normally stimulated by released
    (e) **True**　noradrenaline and which inhibit further transmitter
          release. This is a negative feedback pathway hence there is
          little reflex tachycardia with doxazosin although first dose
          hypotension is a problem; therefore start with a low dose,
          usually at night.

188 (a) **True**　Sodium nitroprusside is valuable in treating hypertensive
    (b) **True**　encephalopathy and in the management of certain types of
    (c) **False**　"shock" when it is combined with positive inotropes.
    (d) **True**　Continuous BP monitoring is essential as it causes
    (e) **True**　profound hypotension. It has a half-life of seconds.

189 (a) **True**　Although generally safe and not contraindicated in asthma
    (b) **True**　and pregnancy, methyldopa is often poorly tolerated.
    (c) **True**　Drowsiness and fatigue may be intolerable when used
    (d) **True**　chronically. It is a well recognized (but uncommon) cause
    (e) **False**　of drug fever and Coombs positive hemolytic anemia.

190 (a) **True**　Many hypertensive patients are successfully treated with a
    (b) **True**　single drug. Diuretics worsen symptoms of bladder neck
    (c) **False**　obstruction, whereas α_1 antagonists improve such
    (d) **False**　symptoms as well as synergizing with ACE inhibitors.
    (e) **True**

191 (a) **True**　– More common in slow acetylators
    (b) **True**　– Fluid retention is also a problem
    (c) **True**　– Worse if on diuretics
    (d) **False**　– May reduce tremor
    (e) **False**　– Rebound hypertension, dry mouth, depression and
            sedation are the main adverse effects

192 The following hypotensive drugs have a potentially deleterious effect on lipid profile:

(a) Thiazide diuretics
(b) β-Blockers
(c) Losartan
(d) Nifedipine
(e) Doxazosin

193 The following drugs are considered to have particular value for the indication named:

(a) Hypertension in a diabetic with albuminuria – trandolapril
(b) Hypertension and ischemic heart disease in a patient with asthma – nifedipine
(c) Acute aortic dissection – sodium nitroprusside
(d) Hypertension in a professional soccer player – atenolol
(e) Imminent eclampsia – hydralazine

194 Management of acute myocardial infarction should usually include (unless contraindicated):

(a) 24% oxygen
(b) Intravenous opiate with an antiemetic
(c) Aspirin
(d) A fibrinolytic drug (e.g. streptokinase)
(e) Lignocaine (lidocaine)

195 The management of unstable angina usually includes:

(a) Aspirin
(b) Glyceryl trinitrate
(c) Intravenous heparin or low molecular weight heparin
(d) Salbutamol
(e) β-Adrenoceptor antagonist

196 Glyceryl trinitrate (GTN):

(a) Relaxes vascular smooth muscle
(b) Is associated with tolerance more commonly with transdermal GTN patches than sublingual GTN
(c) Is volatile
(d) Is relatively more selective for arteriolar than for venous smooth muscle
(e) May relieve the pain of esophageal spasm

192 (a) **True**   The potentially deleterious effects on lipid profile are of
     (b) **True**   unproven clinical significance to date.
     (c) **False**
     (d) **False**
     (e) **False**

193 (a) **True**   The choice of hypotensive drug must be individually
     (b) **True**   tailored to the patient. The first line drugs in
     (c) **True**   uncomplicated hypertension remain a thiazide or a
     (d) **False**   β-blocker in patients without contraindications.
     (e) **True**

194 (a) **False**   The highest concentration of oxygen available should be
     (b) **True**   used unless there is coincident pulmonary disease with
     (c) **True** CO_2 retention. Aspirin and thrombolytic therapy have an
     (d) **True**   additive beneficial effect on reduction of infarct size and
     (e) **False**   improvement in survival. There is evidence of some benefit
                 from early treatment with ACE inhibitors post-infarction in
                 patients with left ventricular dysfunction.

195 (a) **True**   Patients with unstable angina require urgent antiplatelet
     (b) **True**   therapy (aspirin) and urgent admission. Eptifibatide and
     (c) **True**   tirofibran, platelet IIb/IIIa receptor blockers, are used in
     (d) **False**   specialist centers in combination with heparin and aspirin.
     (e) **True**

196 (a) **True**   GTN is generally best used as acute prophylaxis (i.e.
     (b) **True**   immediately before undertaking strenuous activity). The
     (c) **True**   spray has a longer "shelf-life" but is more expensive than
     (d) **False**   the sublingual GTN. GTN is subject to extensive
     (e) **True**   presystemic metabolism if swallowed. Longer acting oral
                 nitrates (e.g. isosorbide mononitrate) are effective as regular
                 prophylactic therapy.

197 Beta-adrenoceptor antagonists:

(a) Increase cardiac tissue cyclic adenosine monophosphate (cAMP)
(b) Competitively antagonize the β-receptor mediated effects of adrenaline and noradrenaline
(c) Non-competitively antagonize several of the actions of thyroxine
(d) Decrease peripheral vascular resistance
(e) Reduce renin secretion

198 The following drugs may reduce the risk of recurrence or death post-myocardial infarction:

(a) Aspirin
(b) β-Blockers
(c) Dexfenfluramine
(d) Sildenafil
(e) Statins

199 Diltiazem is used:

(a) For prophylaxis of angina
(b) To treat hypertension
(c) To treat ventricular tachycardia
(d) To prevent cerebral vasospasm following subarachnoid hemorrhage
(e) To treat left ventricular failure

200 A calcium channel blocker such as amlodipine or nifedipine is preferred to a β-blocker such as atenolol to treat angina in patients who also have:

(a) Chronic bronchitis
(b) Peripheral vascular disease
(c) Heart block
(d) Diabetes
(e) Anxiety

201 Aspirin:

(a) Reduces the risk of stroke in patients with transient ischemic attacks
(b) Predisposes to peptic ulceration
(c) Irreversibly inhibits fatty acid cyclo-oxygenase
(d) Has no effect on bleeding time
(e) Needs to be given twice daily to prevent platelet cyclo-oxygenase resynthesis within the dose interval

197 (a) **False**   β-Blockers slow the heart, are negatively inotropic and
    (b) **True**   reduce arterial blood pressure, are anti-arrhythmic,
    (c) **True**   increase peripheral vascular resistance, reduce plasma
    (d) **False**   renin activity and predispose to bronchoconstriction.
    (e) **True**

198 (a) **True**   Modifiable risk factors should be sought and attended to.
    (b) **True**   ACE inhibitors are recommended for patients with left
    (c) **False**   ventricular dysfunction.
    (d) **False**
    (e) **True**

199 (a) **True**   In addition to hypertension and angina, verapamil is used
    (b) **True**   to treat supraventricular tachycardia. Nimodipine helps
    (c) **False**   prevent cerebral vasospasm and nifedipine is used in
    (d) **False**   Raynaud's syndrome.
    (e) **False**

200 (a) **True**   The commonest side effects of nifedipine and amlodipine
    (b) **True**   are flushing and headache. They have no significant
    (c) **True**   effect on the conduction system of the heart.
    (d) **True**
    (e) **False**

201 (a) **True**   Thromboxane (TX) A$_2$ is the main cyclo-oxygenase product
    (b) **True**   of activated platelets and is proaggregatory and a
    (c) **True**   vasoconstrictor.
    (d) **False**
    (e) **False**

202 Streptokinase:

(a) Is derived from streptococci
(b) Reduces the acute mortality of myocardial infarction only if administered within 4 hours of the onset of chest pain
(c) Is contraindicated if the patient is taking regular non-steroidal anti-inflammatory drug therapy
(d) Is administered by intravenous infusion
(e) Should not be given to patients over the age of 60 years

203 Alteplase:

(a) Is a prodrug that liberates streptokinase
(b) Heparin must not be administered within 24 hours of alteplase infusion
(c) Should only be administered if pulmonary artery pressure can be measured
(d) Is administered via the intramuscular route
(e) Is contraindicated if aspirin has been administered in the last 24 hours

204 The following are relative contraindications to the use of streptokinase in acute myocardial infarction:

(a) Therapy with anistreplase from 5 days to 12 months previously
(b) Stroke due to cerebral thrombosis in the last 6 months
(c) Concurrent hormone replacement therapy for menopausal symptoms
(d) Pulmonary disease with cavitation
(e) Diabetic retinopathy

205 Heparin:

(a) Binds to antithrombin III
(b) Inhibits the action of thrombin
(c) Is monitored in the laboratory by measurement of activated partial thromboplastin time (APTT)
(d) Is less effective in patients with inherited or acquired deficiency of antithrombin III
(e) Is reversed by protamine sulfate

202 (a) **True**   Streptokinase combines with plasminogen to form an
   (b) **False** activator complex that converts remaining free
   (c) **False** plasminogen to plasmin which dissolves fibrin. The
   (d) **True**   potential benefit lessens with delay but the value of
   (e) **False** treatment within 24 hours is well established.

203 (a) **False** Alteplase is a direct-acting plasminogen activator.
   (b) **False** Immediate heparin following alteplase is necessary to
   (c) **False** prevent re-occlusion.
   (d) **False**
   (e) **False**

204 (a) **True**   Immune reactions are important with streptokinase and
   (b) **True**   its prodrug anistreplase. It seems unlikely that mild
   (c) **False** infections such as sore throats reduce its efficacy.
   (d) **True**   "Recent" dental extraction is considered a contraindication.
   (e) **True**

205 (a) **True**   Heparin binds to antithrombin III, the naturally occurring
   (b) **True**   inhibitor of thrombin and of the other serine proteases
   (c) **True**   (factors IXa, Xa and XIa), enormously potentiating its
   (d) **True**   inhibitory action.
   (e) **True**

206 Heparin prophylaxis to prevent deep vein thrombosis/pulmonary embolism in major surgery:

(a) Must be started 1 week before surgery
(b) Is via twice daily intramuscular heparin
(c) Is more likely to be of value in an obese man of 50 than in a slim man of 30
(d) Low molecular weight heparin is an alternative to standard heparin
(e) Concomitant antibiotics are contraindicated

207 The following are recognized adverse effects of heparin therapy:

(a) Osteoporosis
(b) Alopecia
(c) Thrombocytopenia
(d) Diarrhea
(e) Fetal cleft palate

208 The following statements are correct:

(a) In the management of pulmonary embolism heparin is normally administered as an intravenous bolus followed by a continuous infusion
(b) Prophylactic subcutaneous heparin should be monitored by measurement of prothrombin time
(c) Heparin does not affect the thrombin time
(d) Heparin exhibits dose-dependent pharmacokinetics
(e) Immune thrombocytopenia is less common with low molecular weight heparin

209 Warfarin:

(a) Prevents the hepatic synthesis of the vitamin-K dependent coagulation factors II, VII, IX and X
(b) Is structurally closely related to vitamin K
(c) Should initially be given as a subcutaneous loading dose
(d) During life-threatening bleeding can be reversed by vitamin K and factor IX concentrate
(e) Anticoagulant effect is monitored by measurement of the prothrombin time/INR (international normalized ratio)

206 (a) **False**   Prophylactic subcutaneous heparin reduces the risk of
(b) **False**   thromboembolism associated with major surgery. A lower
(c) **True**   concentration of heparin is required to inhibit factor Xa
(d) **True**   early in the cascade than is needed to antagonize the
(e) **False**   actions of thrombin and this provides the rationale for the
use of low dose heparin in prophylaxis. The benefit
normally outweighs the increased risk of bleeding in major
orthopedic surgery.

207 (a) **True**   The commonest adverse effect is bleeding. This can be
(b) **True**   treated by stopping the infusion (if relevant), local
(c) **True**   compression, protamine sulfate and if severe and
(d) **False**   continues in spite of the above, fresh frozen plasma.
(e) **False**

208 (a) **True**   Owing to its short half-life (0.5–2.5 hours), dose-dependent
(b) **False**   kinetics and wide interindividual variation intravenous
(c) **False**   heparin is ideally administered as an infusion with
(d) **True**   monitoring of APTT. Low molecular weight heparin
(e) **True**   (LMWH) is a more specific anticoagulant which is used
prophylactically at low doses and occasionally in patients
who have heparin-induced immune thrombocytopenia. The
standard prophylactic regime is via a once daily
subcutaneous injection and does not require monitoring.
At the doses used to treat deep vein thrombosis and
pulmonary embolism LMWH should not prolong APTT
and may be monitored by factor Xa assay.

209 (a) **True**   Warfarin is the most commonly prescribed oral
(b) **True**   anticoagulant. It usually takes at least 3 days to achieve
(c) **False**   adequate anticoagulation. If more rapid action is required
(d) **True**   intravenous heparin and oral warfarin are used until the
(e) **True**   INR is in the usual therapeutic range (2–3 for most
indications). Heparin only influences the INR if the APTT
> 2.5 the control. The laboratory can allow for this by the *in
vitro* addition of protamine.

210 The following are relative or absolute contraindications to warfarin therapy:

  (a) First trimester of pregnancy
  (b) Prosthetic heart valves
  (c) Space-occupying CNS lesion
  (d) Concurrent digoxin therapy
  (e) G6PD deficiency

211 The following drugs inhibit the metabolism of warfarin:

  (a) Cimetidine
  (b) Fluvoxamine
  (c) St John's wort
  (d) Carbamazepine
  (e) Smoking

212 The following inhibit platelet activation and/or aggregation:

  (a) Warfarin
  (b) Heparin
  (c) Thromboxane A_2
  (d) Prostacyclin (epoprostenol)
  (e) Dipyridamole

213 Prostacyclin (epoprostenol):

  (a) Relaxes pulmonary and systemic vasculature
  (b) Is the principal endogenous prostaglandin of large- and medium-sized blood vessels
  (c) Is an effective anticoagulant
  (d) Is contraindicated in hemodialysis
  (e) Increases diastolic pressure

214 The principal beneficial effect in heart failure of the following drugs is to reduce preload (left ventricular filling pressure):

  (a) Digoxin
  (b) Frusemide (furosemide)
  (c) Dobutamine
  (d) GTN
  (e) Sodium nitroprusside

210 (a) **True**   Other contraindications include active bleeding, blood
    (b) **False**   dyscrasias with hemorrhagic diatheses, dissecting aneurysm
    (c) **True**   of the aorta and recent CNS surgery. Aspirin and warfarin
    (d) **False**   should not be used together routinely, although trials of
    (e) **False**   low dose combination therapy are in progress.

211 (a) **True**   Warfarin has a narrow therapeutic range and steep dose
    (b) **True**   response curve. It is metabolized by CYP_{450}. Cimetidine,
    (c) **False**   an H_2 blocker used to reduce gastric acid production, and
    (d) **False**   fluvoxamine, a SSRI antidepressant, both inhibit CYP_{450}.
    (e) **False**   St John's wort, carbamazepine and smoking induce CYP_{450}.
                      The INR must be monitored to reduce both the risk of
                      bleeding and inadequate anticoagulation.

212 (a) **False**   Thromboxane A_2 is synthesized by activated platelets and
    (b) **True**   acts on platelet receptors to cause further activation and
    (c) **False**   propagation of the aggregate. It also acts on vascular
    (d) **True**   smooth muscle to cause vasoconstriction. Heparin inhibits
    (e) **True**   thrombin, which is a platelet agonist, as well as causing
                      coagulation.

213 (a) **True**   Prostacyclin may be used to prevent coagulation in
    (b) **True**   extracorporeal circuits. It causes flushing, headache,
    (c) **True**   reduced diastolic pressure, increased pulse pressure and
    (d) **False**   usually a reflex tachycardia. Occasionally vagally mediated
    (e) **False**   bradycardia and hypotension occur.

214 (a) **False**   The major influences on preload are blood volume and
    (b) **True**   capacitance vessel tone.
    (c) **False**
    (d) **True**
    (e) **False**

215 The following drugs at standard therapeutic doses aggravate heart failure:

(a) Isosorbide mononitrate
(b) Verapamil
(c) Daunorubicin
(d) Ibuprofen
(e) Bendrofluazide

216 In acute pulmonary edema the following are usually appropriate:

(a) Sublingual nifedipine
(b) Lie the patient supine
(c) Oxygen
(d) Intravenous loop diuretic
(e) Intravenous morphine

217 Intravenous frusemide (furosemide):

(a) Causes natriuresis
(b) Causes kaliuresis
(c) Has an indirect vasodilator effect
(d) Diuresis begins 10–20 minutes after an intravenous dose
(e) High doses are ototoxic

218 Angiotension-converting enzyme (ACE) inhibitors:

(a) Are positive inotropes
(b) Reduce afterload
(c) Reduce preload
(d) May cause cough
(e) Should be given parenterally in acute heart failure

219 Dobutamine:

(a) Is a sympathomimetic amine
(b) Is predominantly a β_1-receptor agonist
(c) Increases blood pressure via vasoconstriction
(d) Should not be given at the same time as loop diuretics
(e) Increases myocardial oxygen consumption

215 (a) **False**   Negative inotropes, direct cardiac toxins (e.g. daunorubicin)
    (b) **True**   and drugs that cause salt retention (e.g. NSAIDs) aggravate
    (c) **True**   heart failure. *Excessive tachycardia* does not allow sufficient
    (d) **True**   time for the ventricle to fill in diastole.
    (e) **False**

216 (a) **False**   In addition to helping relieve the acute anxiety and
    (b) **False**   discomfort associated with acute pulmonary edema opioids
    (c) **True**   dilate capacitance vessels.
    (d) **True**
    (e) **True**

217 (a) **True**   Loop diuretics inhibit $Na^+/K^+/2Cl^-$ cotransport in the thick
    (b) **True**   ascending limb of Henlé's loop.
    (c) **True**
    (d) **True**
    (e) **True**

218 (a) **False**   ACE inhibitors are a major advance in the treatment of
    (b) **True**   cardiac failure acting as arterial and venous vasodilators
    (c) **True**   and prolonging survival.
    (d) **True**
    (e) **False**

219 (a) **True**   Dobutamine is a positive inotrope used predominantly in
    (b) **True**   cardiogenic shock. Hypovolemia must be corrected before
    (c) **False**   its use.
    (d) **False**
    (e) **True**

220 The following drugs can cause sinus tachycardia:

  (a) Esmolol
  (b) Theophylline
  (c) Dobutamine
  (d) Amphetamine
  (e) Digoxin

221 Lignocaine (lidocaine):

  (a) Is a class l b agent that blocks cardiac Na^+ channels, reducing the rate of rise of the cardiac action potential and increasing the effective refractory period
  (b) Is epileptogenic
  (c) Is a positive inotrope
  (d) Is usually administered as an intravenous bolus followed by infusion
  (e) Is the drug of first choice for supraventricular tachycardia

222 The following drugs prolong the QT interval and / or cause torsades de pointes:

  (a) Erythromycin
  (b) Foscarnet
  (c) Pimozide
  (d) Tacrolimus
  (e) Thioridazine

223 The following prolong the QT interval and/or cause torsades de pointes:

  (a) Quinidine
  (b) Disopyramide
  (c) Phenytoin
  (d) Amitriptyline
  (e) Magnesium

224 Amiodarone:

  (a) Is indicated in resistant atrial fibrillation or flutter
  (b) Is effective in preventing recurrent ventricular fibrillation
  (c) Is contraindicated in Wolff–Parkinson–White (WPW) syndrome
  (d) May be given intravenously via a central line
  (e) Prolongs the QT interval

220 (a) **False**   The management of sinus tachycardia is directed to the
    (b) **True**   underlying cause (e.g. pain, anxiety, left ventricular failure,
    (c) **True**   asthma, thyrotoxicosis) and iatrogenic factors. Of calcium
    (d) **True**   antagonists, verapamil causes bradycardia, dihyropyridines
    (e) **False**   can cause reflex tachycardia, and diltiazem seldom causes
                      appreciable changes in heart rate. Esmolol is a β-blocker
                      with a very short duration of action.

221 (a) **True**   Lignocaine has a narrow therapeutic index but is used for
    (b) **True**   the treatment of ventricular tachycardia and fibrillation
    (c) **False**   (post-DC cardioconversion).
    (d) **True**
    (e) **False**

222 (a) **True**
    (b) **True**   – Used for CMV retinitis and AIDS patients
    (c) **True**
    (d) **True**   – An immunosuppressant whose adverse effects include
                     cardiomyopathy
    (e) **True**

223 (a) **True**   A prolonged QT interval predisposes to torsades de pointes,
    (b) **True**   a form of ventricular tachycardia.
    (c) **False**
    (d) **True**
    (e) **False**

224 (a) **True**   Amiodarone, a class III agent, is highly effective in both
    (b) **True**   supraventricular and ventricular arrhythmias. It is not a
    (c) **False**   negative inotrope in contrast to most antiarrhythmic agents.
    (d) **True**
    (e) **True**

225 The following adverse effects are associated with amiodarone:

- (a) Visual disturbances (e.g. colored halos)
- (b) Hyperthyroidism
- (c) Hypothyroidism
- (d) Pulmonary fibrosis
- (e) Photosensitivity

226 Amiodarone:

- (a) Is highly lipid soluble
- (b) Has an apparent volume of distribution of approximately 5000 litres
- (c) Is predominantly eliminated by the kidney
- (d) Accumulates in the heart
- (e) Has a half-life of 28–45 days

227 Sotalol:

- (a) Is effective in supraventricular and ventricular arrhythmias
- (b) Is not effective when given by mouth
- (c) The dose should be reduced in renal impairment
- (d) May cause torsades de pointes
- (e) Is a less potent negative inotrope than amiodarone

228 Intravenous verapamil:

- (a) May terminate supraventricular tachycardia
- (b) Must not be given to patients receiving β-blockers
- (c) Reduces digoxin excretion
- (d) One must delay DC cardioversion at least 2 hours after a dose
- (e) Shortens the PR interval

229 Adenosine:

- (a) Is used to terminate ventricular tachycardia
- (b) Is contraindicated in regular broad complex tachycardia
- (c) Dilates bronchial smooth muscle
- (d) Is associated with chest pain
- (e) Circulatory effects last 20–30 seconds

225 (a) **True**   Adverse effects are many and varied and are common when
     (b) **True**   plasma amiodarone concentration exceeds 2.5 mg/L.
     (c) **True**   Most are reversible on stopping treatment, but this is not
     (d) **True**   true of pulmonary fibrosis.
     (e) **True**

226 (a) **True**   Amiodarone is highly protein bound and is slowly excreted
     (b) **True**   by the liver. Antiarrhythmic activity may persist for several
     (c) **False**   months after stopping treatment.
     (d) **True**
     (e) **True**

227 (a) **True**   Sotalol is a β-adrenoreceptor antagonist (class ll) with
     (b) **False**   additional class III antiarrhythmic activity.
     (c) **True**
     (d) **True**
     (e) **False**

228 (a) **True**   Verapamil slows intracardiac conduction affecting in
     (b) **True**   particular the AV node but also the SA node. It is a potent
     (c) **True**   negative inotrope. It should be avoided in WPW as it can
     (d) **False**   increase conduction through an accessory pathway.
     (e) **False**

229 (a) **False**   Adenosine is used to terminate supraventricular
     (b) **False**   tachycardia (SVT). It is particularly useful diagnostically in
     (c) **False**   patients with regular broad complex tachycardia which is
     (d) **True**   suspected of being SVT with aberrant conduction. If
     (e) **True**   adenosine terminates the bradycardia the AV node is
                 involved.

230 Digoxin:

(a) Reduces the ventricular rate in atrial fibrillation
(b) Is contraindicated in second degree heart block
(c) Is the treatment of choice in atrial fibrillation in a patient with WPW
(d) Induced arrhythmias may be terminated by magnesium
(e) 80% of administered digoxin is excreted unchanged in the bile

231 A 70-year-old woman has recurrent, symptomatic ventricular tachycardia following an acute myocardial infarction in spite of DC conversion and lignocaine. The following may be effective:

(a) Amiodarone
(b) Bretylium
(c) Verapamil
(d) Adenosine
(e) Isoprenaline

232 The following are indications for transvenous pacing:

(a) Symptomatic sinus bradycardia post inferior myocardial infarction
(b) First degree heart block post-inferior myocardial infarction
(c) A heart rate of 34 bpm at rest in an athlete with second degree (Mobitz type 1) heart block
(d) Asymptomatic congenital complete heart block
(e) Blackouts associated with bradycardia in sick sinus syndrome

233 The following arrhythmias are correctly paired with their first line treatment:

(a) Ventricular fibrillation – synchronized DC cardioversion
(b) Ventricular fibrillation – unsynchronized DC cardioversion
(c) Ventricular tachycardia post myocardial infarction – propranolol
(d) Rapid atrial fibrillation – flecainide
(e) Drug-induced torsades de pointes – disopyramide

230 (a) **True** The main use of digoxin as an antiarrhythmic is to control
    (b) **True** the ventricular rate (and hence improve cardiac output) in
    (c) **False** patients with atrial fibrillation. Drugs causing hypokalemia
    (d) **True** aggravate digoxin toxicity.
    (e) **False**

231 (a) **True** Isoprenaline, a β-agonist, is likely to be arrhythmogenic
    (b) **True** and will increase myocardial oxygen consumption.
    (c) **False** Verapamil is a potent negative inotrope and is only effective
    (d) **False** in supra-ventricular tachycardia.
    (e) **False**

232 (a) **False** Bradycardia and first degree heart block are common post
    (b) **False** inferior myocardial infarction. If the bradycardia causes
    (c) **False** symptoms 0.6 mg atropine IV is usually effective.
    (d) **False**
    (e) **True**

233 (a) **False** If causing immediate cardiovascular embarrassment, DC
    (b) **True** cardioversion is indicated in ventricular tachycardia. Other
    (c) **False** wise, if intravenous lignocaine is ineffective, or oral
    (d) **False** prophylaxis is required, amiodarone may be used.
    (e) **False** Intravenous magnesium sulfate has been recommended for
                   torsades de pointes. It also has a major role in eclampsia for
                   the prevention of recurrent seizures.

CHAPTER FIVE

Respiratory System

234 The following should be administered to an otherwise healthy 27-year-old male with acute severe asthma:

(a) Intravenous midazolam
(b) Nebulized salbutamol
(c) Intravenous corticosteroids
(d) Nebulized sodium cromoglycate
(e) Continuous high percentage oxygen (Fio_2 35–40%)

235 β_2-Agonists (e.g. salbutamol, terbutaline):

(a) Relax bronchial smooth muscle
(b) Inhibit release of mast cell and other inflammatory mediators
(c) Reduce heart rate
(d) Cause pulmonary vasoconstriction
(e) Decrease intracellular cyclic adenosine monophosphate (cAMP)

236 Properties of salmeterol include:

(a) Tremor
(b) Exacerbation of atrial arrhythmias
(c) Hyperkalemia
(d) Prolonged pharmacodynamic effects allowing twice daily dosing
(e) Seizures

237 Zileuton (a 5'-lipoxygenase inhibitor available in the USA):

(a) Is contraindicated in patients with aspirin induced asthma
(b) Is used in the maintenance treatment of asthma and not in acute attacks
(c) Reduces concentration of leukotrienes
(d) Inhibits warfarin metabolism
(e) Shows tachyphylaxis in its efficacy

234 (a) **False**   Never give sedatives in acute asthma. Intravenous fluids are
    (b) **True**   administered to correct/prevent dehydration. Antibiotics
    (c) **True**   are administered if there is history/signs of infection.
    (d) **False**   Refractory cases require intravenous β_2-agonist
    (e) **True**   (salbutamol) or theophylline. If these are inadequate,
                    intermittent positive pressure ventilation is required.
                    Nebulized cromoglycate is not effective acutely.

235 (a) **True** β_2-Agonists stimulate the β_2-receptor which via G-proteins
    (b) **True**   increases adenylyl cyclase activity and increases
    (c) **False**   intracellular cAMP. They cause a tachycardia and
    (d) **False**   vasodilatation.
    (e) **False**

236 (a) **True** β_2-Agonists are generally well tolerated when given by
    (b) **True**   inhalation. Salmeterol, a long-acting β_2-agonist, is inhaled
    (c) **False**   twice daily and reduces the need for shorter acting agents
    (d) **True**   and possibly the dose of inhaled steroids. (β-Agonists cause
    (e) **False**   hypokalaemia.)

237 (a) **False**   It inhibits the 5'-lipoxygenase enzyme that is involved in
    (b) **True**   synthesis of all leukotrienes. Therefore as aspirin is believed
    (c) **True**   to exacerbate asthma by diverting arachidonic acid towards
    (d) **True**   leukotriene metabolism, zileuton will be of benefit to
    (e) **False**   patients with aspirin induced asthma. It inhibits the CYP_{450}
                    involved in warfarin metabolism.

238 Ipratropium bromide:

(a) Is administered intravenously
(b) Causes bronchodilatation because of its antagonistic effects at the cholinergic M_2/M_3 receptors
(c) Has a more rapid onset of bronchodilatation than β_2-agonists
(d) Has a bitter taste
(e) May precipitate glaucoma in high doses

239 Theophylline:

(a) Is usually administered via a metered dose inhaler (MDI)
(b) Inhibits the catabolism of cAMP by phosphodiesterase
(c) Causes concentration related increases in FEV_1 at plasma concentrations between 10 and 20 mg/L
(d) Antagonizes adenosine at A_2-receptors
(e) Is a metabolite of salmeterol.

240 Adverse effects associated with the use of theophylline include:

(a) Cardiac arrhythmias
(b) Convulsions
(c) Oral candidiasis
(d) Headache
(e) Nausea and vomiting

238 (a) **False**   Inhaled antimuscarinic drugs such as ipratropium and
    (b) **True**   oxitropium are effective as acute and maintenance therapy
    (c) **False**   in asthma. Its action is slower in onset than β_2-agonists.
    (d) **True**   High doses usually via a nebulizer may precipitate acute
    (e) **True**   glaucoma or urinary retention.

239 (a) **False**   Theophylline is administered via the oral route (usually in
    (b) **True**   slow release formulations) or the intravenous route (as
    (c) **True**   aminophylline a combination of theophylline and ethylene
    (d) **True**   diamine) or rarely, via the rectal route. It is metabolized
    (e) **False**   mainly by CYP1A2 in the liver.

240 (a) **True**   Theophylline has a narrow therapeutic index and its
    (b) **True**   pharmacokinetics show considerable interindividual
    (c) **False**   variation. Because of liver metabolism it is prone to a
    (d) **True**   number of drug–drug interactions which may lead to
    (e) **True**   toxicity (see Table 3 below). Its main side effects are
                     gastrointestinal, cardiovascular and CNS.

Table 3 Factors influencing theophylline clearance

Factors decreasing theophylline clearance and suggested initial *dose adjustment (assuming normal dose is 100%)	Factors increasing theophylline clearance and suggested initial *dose adjustment (assuming normal dose is 100%)
Congestive cardiac failure (40%)	Hyperthyroidism (150%)
Hepatic disease, cirrhosis (40%)	Marijuana (150%)
Neonates (60%)	Smoking (150%)
Pneumonia (70%)	Charcoal barbecued meat (130%)
Old age (80%)	
Drugs	Drugs
Azole-antifungals (e.g. ketoconazole, etc.) (50%)	Carbamazepine (150%)
Cimetidine (50%)	Phenytoin (150%)
Fluoroquinolones (e.g. ciprofloxacin) (50%)	Rifampicin (150%)
Chloramphenicol (75%)	High protein, low carbohydrate diet (150%)
Erythromycin (75%)	Ethanol (chronic) (120%)
Flu vaccine and interferon (75%)	
Propranolol (70%)	

* Subsequent does adjustment to be made in the light of plasma concentration monitoring, which should be carried out more frequently in the circumstances listed. The suggested adjustments are obviously very approximate, and depend on the extent of exposure to the various agents.

241 The following decrease the clearance of theophylline:

(a) Congestive cardiac failure
(b) Cirrhosis
(c) Marijuana
(d) Concurrent ciprofloxacin therapy
(e) Smoking

242 In acute severe asthma hydrocortisone:

(a) Is usually given via the intravenous route
(b) Subjective improvement following steroid administration takes 30–60 minutes
(c) Is contraindicated in growing children
(d) Is contraindicated in pregnancy
(e) Should not be administered until at least two doses of nebulized salbutamol have been administered without significant evidence of sustained bronchodilatation

243 Administration of beclomethasone via a metered dose inhaler:

(a) Allows reduction in the maintenance dose of oral prednisolone in chronic asthma
(b) More of the dose is swallowed than enters the lungs
(c) Does not cause hypothalamo-pituitary-adrenal suppression at a dose of 2000 µg/day
(d) Has a lower systemic bioavailability than fluticasone
(e) In children, causes reversible inhibition of long bone growth at high doses

244 Inhaled sodium cromoglycate:

(a) Is effective in alleviating an acute episode of allergic asthma
(b) Has no benefit in preventing exercise induced bronchospasm
(c) Prevents antigen–antibody combination
(d) Inhibits mediator release from mast cells
(e) Causes cardiac arrhythmias by prolonging the QTc

241 (a) **True**
    (b) **True**
    (c) **False** – Marijuana increases theophylline clearance
    (d) **True**
    (e) **False**

242 (a) **True**   Objective improvement does not occur until 6 hours and is
    (b) **False**   maximal 13 hours after the start of intravenous
    (c) **False**   corticosteroid treatment in asthma. This delay is due to the
    (d) **False**   pharmacodynamics of glucocorticoids which work via
    (e) **False**   modifying transcription of certain genes and thus affecting
    their protein synthesis. They should be administered early
    in acute asthma.

243 (a) **True**   Systemic adverse events are rarely significant with inhaled
    (b) **True**   glucocorticoids unless the dose exceeds e.g 1600 µg of
    (c) **False**   beclomethasone or its equivalent. They are invaluable in
    (d) **False**   the prophylaxis of asthma and have been shown to reduce
    (e) **True**   asthma deaths.

244 (a) **False**   Sodium cromoglycate is administered by inhalation of a
    (b) **False**   powder. Used prophylactically it can prevent type I and
    (c) **False**   type III allergic reactions and exercise induced asthma. It is
    (d) **True**   very safe although approximately 1:10 000 experience
    (e) **False**   cough or hoarseness.

245 Montelukast:

(a) Is a competitive antagonist at the Cys LT_1 receptor
(b) Can be given orally
(c) Is usually taken once daily at bedtime
(d) May be associated with Churg–Strauss syndrome
(e) Is not beneficial to patients with antigen induced asthma

246 The following drugs can produce pulmonary fibrosis:

(a) Methotrexate
(b) Bleomycin
(c) Busulphan
(d) Captopril
(e) Amiodarone

247 Pulmonary eosinophilia is caused by the following drugs:

(a) Methysergide
(b) Aspirin
(c) Nitrofurantoin
(d) Carmustine (BCNU)
(e) Sulfasalazine

248 The following agents if given to an asthmatic can cause catastrophic bronchospasm

(a) Carvedilol
(b) Losartan
(c) Adenosine
(d) Lignocaine (lidocaine)
(e) Bethanecol

249 The following drugs are used as "standard of care" when treating a patient with type-II respiratory failure:

(a) 24–28% oxygen
(b) Doxapram
(c) Salbutamol
(d) Methylprednisolone
(e) Dantrolene

245 (a) **True**   It is a potent, oral, once daily inhibitor of cysteinyl
    (b) **True**   leukotrienes at the Cys LT$_1$ receptor. Thus its main action is
    (c) **True**   to antagonize the potent pro-inflammatory effects of
    (d) **True**   leukotrienes It causes about a 5–10% increase in baseline
    (e) **False**   FEV$_1$ but this takes about 1 hour to manifest. About 5% of
                    patients develop a reversible transaminitis.

246 (a) **True**   Several cytotoxics particularly if given with or following
    (b) **True**   radiation cause a severe pulmonary fibrosis that may not be
    (c) **True**   reversible. Captopril (as are all ACE inhibitors) is associated
    (d) **False**   with a dose-dependent chronic dry cough thought to be
    (e) **True**   related to bradykinin accumulation.

247 (a) **False**   Methysergide causes retroperitoneal fibrosis. Aspirin
    (b) **True**   (and nitrofurantoin, imipramine, isoniazid, penicillins,
    (c) **True**   sulfonamides and streptomycin) has been associated
    (d) **False**   with pulmonary eosinophilia. Carmustine causes
    (e) **True**   pulmonary fibrosis.

248 (a) **True**   – Carvedilol is a non-selective β-blocker whose indications
                    include hypertension angina and as adjunct to other
                    agents, symptomatic chronic heart failure. The initial dose
                    for this indication is ¼ of the other indications
    (b) **False**
    (c) **True**   – Adenosine causes bronchoconstriction by stimulating
                    adenosine receptors
    (d) **False**
    (e) **True**   – Bethanecol and carbachol are acetylcholine analogs and
                    increase cholinergic (parasympathetic) tone

249 (a) **True**   – Use low FiO$_2$ and titrate upwards based on blood gas
                    response/clinical response
    (b) **False**   – Analeptics are no longer used unless mechanical ventilation
                    is unavailable or contraindicated
    (c) **True**
    (d) **True**
    (e) **False**   – Dantrolene is a muscle relaxant; this would worsen
                    respiratory failure

CHAPTER SIX

Alimentary System

250 The following stimulate gastric acid secretion:

   (a) Vagal stimulation
   (b) Gastrin
   (c) Acetylcholine stimulation of the M_1-receptor
   (d) Histamine stimulation of the H_2-receptor
   (e) Increased intracellular cAMP

250 (a) **True**
    (b) **True**
    (c) **True**
    (d) **True**
    (e) **True**

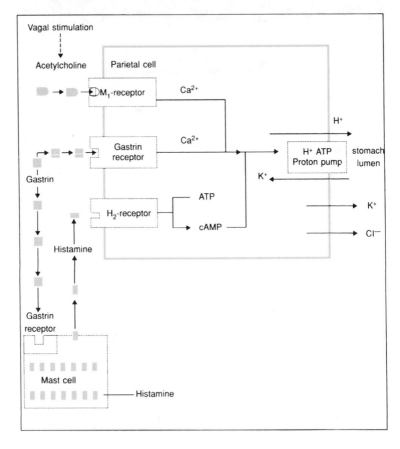

Fig. 2 Mechanisms regulating hydrochloric acid secretion. Ca^{2+}, calcium; ATP, adenosine triphosphate; cAMP, cyclic adenosine monophosphate; K^+, potassium; Cl^-, chloride

251 Prostaglandin E$_2$:

    (a) Is the principal prostaglandin synthesized in the stomach

    (b) Stimulates gastric acid secretion

    (c) Causes vasoconstriction of submucosal blood vessels

    (d) Biosynthesis is inhibited by aspirin

    (e) Biosynthesis is inhibited by rectal indomethacin

252 *Helicobacter pylori:*

    (a) Is strongly linked to the development of carcinoma of the colon

    (b) Is a bacterium that is strongly linked to the development and recurrence of peptic ulcer disease

    (c) Is usually found in the gastric antrum

    (d) Is uncommon in asymptomatic patients

    (e) Colonization of the stomach is inhibited by corticosteroids

253 The following accelerate healing in gastric ulcers:

    (a) Diclofenac

    (b) Stopping smoking

    (c) Corticosteroids

    (d) Cimetidine

    (e) Sucralfate

254 Antacids:

    (a) Large doses heal gastric ulcers more frequently than duodenal ulcers

    (b) Standard doses reduce gastric acidity for approximately 4 hours

    (c) Magnesium salts tend to cause diarrhea

    (d) Aluminum salts tend to cause a diuresis

    (e) Magnesium and aluminum salts reduce the rate and extent of absorption of phenytoin

255 Cimetidine therapy is associated with:

    (a) Transient increase in serum prolactin

    (b) Irreversible gynecomastia

    (c) Mental confusion in the elderly

    (d) Asystole after rapid intravenous injection

    (e) Reversible rise in serum creatinine

251 (a) **True**   Prostaglandin E_2 is an important gastroprotective
    (b) **False**   mediator. It inhibits secretion of acid, promotes secretion
    (c) **False**   of protective mucus and causes vasodilation of submucosal
    (d) **True**   blood vessels.
    (e) **True**

252 (a) **False**   *Helicobacter pylori is* strongly linked to the development and
    (b) **True**   recurrence of duodenal ulcer. Possible linkage to gastric
    (c) **True**   carcinoma is under investigation.
    (d) **False**
    (e) **False**

253 (a) **False** – NSAID, ulcerogenic
    (b) **True** – More effective in preventing recurrence of duodenal ulcers
                than H_2-blockers
    (c) **False** – Ulcerogenic
    (d) **True** – H_2-blocker
    (e) **True**

254 (a) **False**   Antacids produce prompt but transient pain relief in
    (b) **False**   patients with peptic ulceration. Aluminum salts cause
    (c) **True**   constipation.
    (d) **False**
    (e) **True**

255 (a) **True**   Chronic cimetidine therapy causes reversible gynecomastia
    (b) **False**   in 0.11–0.2% of patients. It is generally well tolerated.
    (c) **True**
    (d) **True**
    (e) **True**

256 Eradication of *H. pylori* following a positive breath test is
recommended in the following situations:

   (a) Duodenal ulcer
   (b) Gastric ulcer
   (c) Patients requring long-term proton pump inhibitor treatment
   (d) Severe gastritis
   (e) Mucosa associated lymphoid tissue lymphoma

257 In comparison to cimetidine, ranitidine:

   (a) Does not bind to androgen receptors
   (b) Is less likely to cause gynecomastia
   (c) Penetrates the blood–brain barrier to a lesser extent
   (d) Is not available for parenteral use
   (e) Has a lower affinity for cytochrome P_{450}

258 Omeprazole:

   (a) Is an irreversible inhibitor of the hydrogen/potassium adenosine
       triphosphatase locus of the gastric parietal cell
   (b) Reduces gastric acid secretion
   (c) Is the drug of choice in Zollinger–Ellison syndrome
   (d) Has a plasma half-life of approximately 1 hour
   (e) Requires dose reduction in renal failure

259 Omeprazole enhances the effects of the following drugs through
inhibition of drug metabolism:

   (a) Atenolol
   (b) Amoxycillin
   (c) Captopril
   (d) Warfarin
   (e) Phenytoin

260 Problems associated with proton pump inhbitors include:

   (a) Masking symptoms of gastric cancer
   (b) Diarrhea, nausea and vomiting
   (c) Increased risk of gastrointestinal infection
   (d) Headache
   (e) Prolonged QT interval on ECG

256 (a) **True**   Eradication should be confirmed, preferably by urea breath
    (b) **True**   test at a minimum of 4 weeks post-treatment.
    (c) **True**
    (d) **True**
    (e) **True**

257 (a) **True**   All the H$_2$-receptor blockers currently available in the UK
    (b) **True**   are effective in peptic ulceration and are well tolerated.
    (c) **True**   There is most experience with cimetidine and ranitidine.
    (d) **False**
    (e) **True**

258 (a) **True**   Omeprazole, a proton pump inhibitor, is most effective in
    (b) **True**   reducing gastric secretion and in spite of its short half-life
    (c) **True**   only has to be administered once daily since it acts
    (d) **True**   irreversibly.
    (e) **False**

259 (a) **False**   For drugs such as phenytoin and warfarin which have a
    (b) **False**   narrow therapeutic index this is clinically significant.
    (c) **False**
    (d) **True**
    (e) **True**

260 (a) **True**   There are currently four proton pump inhibitors licensed in
    (b) **True**   the UK: omeprazole, lansoprazole, pantoprazole and
    (c) **True**   rabeprazole.
    (d) **True**
    (e) **False**

261 Misoprostol:

   (a) Is a synthetic analog of prostaglandin E

   (b) Inhibits cyclo-oxygenase

   (c) Causes vasodilatation in the submucosa

   (d) Is rapidly and nearly completely absorbed

   (e) Is contraindicated in pregnancy

262 Bismuth chelate:

   (a) Precipitates at acid pH

   (b) Stimulates mucus production

   (c) Has a direct toxic effect on *Helicobacter pylori*

   (d) Causes pale stools

   (e) Causes nausea

263 Sucralfate:

   (a) Requires systemic absorption for anti-ulcer activity

   (b) Contains aluminum

   (c) Is effective in healing gastric ulcers

   (d) Is contraindicated in pregnancy

   (e) Is associated with constipation

264 The following drugs are used to prevent motion sickness:

   (a) Hyoscine

   (b) Promethazine

   (c) Cinnarizine

   (d) Metoclopramide

   (e) Chlorpromazine

265 Cyclizine:

   (a) Is a dopamine receptor antagonist

   (b) Is effective in morphine-induced vomiting

   (c) Is a proven teratogen

   (d) Causes dry mouth

   (e) Causes drowsiness

261 (a) **True** Misoprostol inhibits gastric acid secretion, causes
(b) **False** vasodilatation in the submucosa and stimulates
(c) **True** production of protective mucus. It contracts uterine muscle
(d) **True** and causes abortion.
(e) **True**

262 (a) **True** Several studies show bismuth chelate to be as active as
(b) **True** cimetidine in the healing of duodenal and gastric ulcers
(c) **True** after 4–8 weeks of treatment. It is, however, associated with
(d) **False** frequent minor adverse effects. It is a part of "triple
(e) **True** therapy" for the eradication of *H. pylori*.

263 (a) **False** Sucralfate, a basic aluminum salt, becomes a sticky
(b) **True** adherent paste in the presence of acid which retains antacid
(c) **True** efficacy and apparently coats the floor of ulcer craters.
(d) **False**
(e) **True**

264 (a) **True** – Muscarinic antagonist; NB: anticholinergic side effects
(b) **True** – H_1-blocker minor anti-muscarinic action
(c) **True** – H_1-blocker minor anti-muscarinic action
(d) **False** – Dopamine receptor antagonist
(e) **False** – Chlorpromazine is not used for motion sickness

265 (a) **False** – H_1-blocker with additional anti-muscarinic actions
(b) **True**
(c) **False**
(d) **True**
(e) **True**

266 Metoclopramide:

(a) Is most effective in centrally mediated vomiting
(b) Is ineffective in drug-induced nausea
(c) Increases the rate of gastric emptying
(d) Should be avoided for 3–4 days following gastrointestinal surgery
(e) High doses block 5HT$_3$ receptors

267 Acute dystonic reactions related to metoclopramide:

(a) Occur in approximately 10% of patients
(b) Include trismus
(c) Are more common in males
(d) Can be treated with benztropine
(e) Can be treated with diazepam

268 Ondansetron:

(a) Is a phenothiazine
(b) Is not absorbed after oral administration
(c) Is effective in preventing nausea and vomiting due to cancer chemotherapy and radiotherapy
(d) Is ineffective in ciplastin-induced nausea
(e) 1% of patients have dystonic reactions

269 In ulcerative colitis:

(a) Intravenous hydrocortisone is of proven value in the treatment of acute colitis
(b) Oral corticosteroids are first line for maintenance treatment
(c) Localized rectal disease often responds to prednisolone enemas/ suppositories
(d) In severe colitis codeine should be used
(e) Fiber is contraindicated

270 Sulfasalazine:

(a) Is a prodrug
(b) Is used for maintenance treatment of ulcerative colitis
(c) Is not effective in small bowel Crohn's disease
(d) Should be avoided in G6PD deficiency
(e) Inhibits directly the proinflammatory mediator, TNF

266 (a) **False** – Relatively ineffective in motion sickness and other forms of centrally mediated vomiting
(b) **False**
(c) **True** – Increases the rate of absorption of oral drugs
(d) **True**
(e) **True** – Effective in some patients in preventing cisplatin-induced nausea and vomiting

267 (a) **False** – About 1%
(b) **True** – Also akathisia, oculogyric crises, torticollis and opisthotonos
(c) **False** – Commoner in females and the young
(d) **True** Domperidone, another dopamine-receptor antagonist, does
(e) **True** not cross the blood–brain barrier and rarely causes extrapyramidal symptoms. It is more expensive than metoclopramide.

268 (a) **False** – Ondansetron is a highly selective $5HT_3$-receptor antagonist
(b) **False** – Is used both orally and intravenously
(c) **True**
(d) **False**
(e) **False** – Causes constipation

269 (a) **True** – Correction of dehydration, nutritional and electrolyte imbalance are life-saving
(b) **False** – Because of side effects
(c) **True** – Some systemic absorption may occur
(d) **False** – May precipitate paralytic ileus and megacolon
(e) **False** – A high fiber diet and bulk-forming drugs are useful in adjusting fecal consistency

270 (a) **True** – Broken down to 5-aminosalicylate and sulfapyridine
(b) **True**
(c) **True**
(d) **True**
(e) **False** – Infliximab has been introduced recently for the treatment of severe active Crohn's disease refractory to corticosteroid or immunosuppressant therapy. It is a monoclonal antibody which inhibits tumor necrosis factor (TNF)

271 Adverse effects associated with sulfasalazine include:

   (a) Blood dyscrasias
   (b) Oligospermia
   (c) Stevens–Johnson syndrome
   (d) SLE-like syndrome
   (e) Hepatitis

272 Mesalazine:

   (a) Is a prodrug consisting of a dimer of two 5-aminosalicylic acid molecules
   (b) Dissolves at the pH found in the terminal ileum and colon
   (c) Is contraindicated in sulfonamide hypersensitivity
   (d) Is associated with oligospermia
   (e) Is associated with interstitial nephritis

273 The following drugs cause constipation:

   (a) Amiodarone
   (b) Amitriptyline
   (c) Amoxycillin
   (d) Misoprostol
   (e) Metformin

274 Lactulose:

   (a) Is a chemical stimulant to the colon
   (b) Produces its effect 10–12 hours after an oral dose
   (c) Requires colonic bacteria for activity
   (d) Should not be administered concurrently with bran
   (e) Is contraindicated in liver failure

275 Loperamide:

   (a) Decreases intestinal transit time
   (b) Increases bulk of gut contents
   (c) Requires systemic absorption for activity on the bowel
   (d) Causes pupil constriction
   (e) Causes hypersalivation

271 (a) **True**   Adverse effects are more common in slow acetlylators.
    (b) **True**
    (c) **True**
    (d) **True**
    (e) **True**

272 (a) **False** – This describes olsalazine
    (b) **True**
    (c) **False** – But is contraindicated in salicylate hypersensitivity
    (d) **False**
    (e) **True** – Contraindicated in renal impairment

273 (a) **True**   The cause of any change in bowel habit should be
    (b) **True**   determined before laxatives are used.
    (c) **False**
    (d) **False**
    (e) **False**

274 (a) **False**   Lactulose is a disaccharide which is broken down in the
    (b) **False**   colon by bacteria to unabsorbed organic anions which
    (c) **True**   retain fluid in the gut lumen.
    (d) **False**
    (e) **False**

275 (a) **False**   See *TCP*, Chapter 33, p. 380. Loperamide rarely causes CNS
    (b) **False**   effects. However, co-administration with quinidine, a
    (c) **False**   known inhibitor of the P-glycoprotein transmembrane
    (d) **False**   pump, is associated with respiratory depression
    (e) **False**   independent of changes in plasma concentration indicating
                     increased CNS penetration.

276 Treatment of hepatic encephalopathy includes:

    (a) Dietary protein restriction
    (b) Emptying the lower bowel
    (c) Oral lactulose
    (d) Prophylactic vitamin K
    (e) Oral methionine

277 The emergency drug therapy of portal hypertension and esophageal varices may include:

    (a) Vasopressin
    (b) Chenodeoxycholic acid
    (c) Calcitonin
    (d) Octreotide
    (e) lsoprenaline

278 The following drugs are associated with cholestatic jaundice/hepatitis:

    (a) Ondansetron
    (b) Methotrexate
    (c) Synthetic estrogens
    (d) Chlorpromazine
    (e) Rifampicin

279 The long-term efficacy and safety of the following drugs in reducing obesity has been established:

    (a) Thyroxine
    (b) Diethylpropion
    (c) Thiazide diuretics
    (d) Pizotifen
    (e) Mazindol

276 (a) **True** See *TCP*, Chapter 33, pp. 383–4.
    (b) **True**
    (c) **True**
    (d) **True**
    (e) **False**

277 (a) **True** See *TCP*, Chapter 33, p. 384.
    (b) **False**
    (c) **False**
    (d) **True**
    (e) **False**

278 (a) **False** – Usually mild and asymptomatic increase in transaminases
    (b) **False** – Hepatic fibrosis/cirrhosis
    (c) **True** – Rare now low dose estrogens are more commonly prescribed
    (d) **True** – Associated with fever, abdominal pain and pruritus
    (e) **True** – Usually transient

279 (a) **False** – Dangerous and irrational in euthyroid patients
    (b) **False** – Related to amphetamine – abuse potential
    (c) **False** – Transient weight loss secondary to fluid loss
    (d) **False** – Inhibits $5HT_2$-receptors, increases appetite and causes weight gain
    (e) **False** – Long-term efficacy not established

CHAPTER SEVEN

Endocrine System

280 In young insulin-dependent diabetic (type 1 diabetic) patients:

(a) There is good evidence that improved diabetic control reduces the incidence of microvascular complications
(b) Blood glucose monitoring should be performed at home
(c) Once-daily subcutaneous insulin usually provides acceptable control
(d) The dietary carbohydrate content should be 45–55% of total calories
(e) A fiber-rich diet reduces peak plasma glucose after meals and reduces insulin requirements

281 Recombinant human insulin in diabetes mellitus:

(a) Never produces allergic reactions
(b) The effective dose may be less than animal insulin
(c) Patients are less aware of hypoglycemia
(d) Should not be given intravenously
(e) Is not of any value in type 2 diabetes mellitus

282 A 17-year-old woman is admitted comatose with diabetic ketoacidosis. The following is accepted as "standard of care":

(a) Administer 500 mL of 0.9% saline in the first 2 hours
(b) Bladder catheterization
(c) Administer subcutaneous insulin 0.1 unit/kg/hour
(d) Administer 8.4% sodium bicarbonate intravenously if the arterial pH is between 7.2 and 7.3
(e) Aspiration of the stomach

280 (a) **True**   In IDDM, in addition to tight diabetic control which can
    (b) **True**   usually be achieved by education and insulin three times
    (c) **False** daily plus diet, there must be regular screening for
    (d) **True**   microvascular complications. Laser therapy of early
    (e) **True**   proliferative retinopathy prevents blindness.

281 (a) **False** – But are much less common than with animal insulin
    (b) **True** – Possibly due to fewer blocking antibodies
    (c) **False** – Initial fears unfounded following double blind studies
    (d) **False**
    (e) **False** – If target glucose values in type 2 diabetes mellitus are not
                    achieved with diet and oral glucose lowering agents, insulin
                    is used

282 (a) **False** – 1.5–2 litres over the first 2 hours
    (b) **True** – Helps in accurate monitoring of urine output. A central
                    venous pressure line also aids fluid management
    (c) **False** – Give intravenous short acting insulin via syringe pump
    (d) **False** – May worsen intracellular and cerebrospinal acidemia
    (e) **True** – Gastric stasis is common and inhalation of vomit can be
                    fatal. Insertion of a cuffed endotracheal tube may be
                    necessary before nasogastric aspiration depending on the
                    patient's conscious level

283 Sulfonylureas:

(a) Are used in obese diabetics who show a tendency to ketosis
(b) Improve symptoms of polyuria and polydipsia
(c) Have been proven to reduce the vascular complications of non-insulin dependent diabetes mellitus (NIDDM – type II diabetics)
(d) Require functioning β-cells for a hypoglycemic effect
(e) Are usually administered once daily at bed time

284 Gliclazide:

(a) Should never be combined with pioglitazone
(b) Has a shorter half-life than chlorpropamide
(c) Hypoglycemia can be reversed by intramuscular glucagon
(d) Should not be prescribed concurrently with metformin
(e) Stimulates appetite

285 Metformin, a biguanide:

(a) May cause lactic acidosis
(b) Is particularly useful in alcoholic diabetic patients
(c) Causes hypoglycemia in non-diabetic patients
(d) Should be discontinued before major elective surgery
(e) Causes anorexia and weight loss

286 Carbimazole:

(a) Decreases thyroid hormone synthesis
(b) Inhibits the peripheral conversion of T_4 to the more active T_3
(c) Should be stopped immediately if a rash develops
(d) Has an active metabolite
(e) Is associated with neutropenia

287 The following may cause hypercalcemia:

(a) Plicamycin
(b) Calcitonin
(c) Bisphosphonates
(d) 1-α calcidol
(e) Thiazide diuretics

283 (a) **False**
  (b) **True**
  (c) **False** – Early and effective treatment of hypertension does reduce the macro- and microvascular complications of diabetes
  (d) **True** – Increase plasma insulin concentrations
  (e) **False** – Most commonly as a single dose with breakfast

284 (a) **False** – Pioglitazone, which reduces the body's resistance to insulin, may be combined with sulfonylureas in patients intolerant to metformin. Liver toxicity is a concern and liver function rests should be checked before and during treatment
  (b) **True**
  (c) **True** – A useful alternative to intravenous glucose if the patient is unable to take glucose orally and venous access is impractical (e.g. in the home) or unavailable
  (d) **False**
  (e) **True** – cf. metformin

285 (a) **True**   Metformin is useful in obese patients with NIDDM
  (b) **False**   uncontrolled by diet and a sulfonylurea. The anorexia is
  (c) **False**   useful in obese diabetic patients. Lactic acidosis is the most
  (d) **True**   sinister adverse effect and has a high mortality. Metformin
  (e) **True**   is contraindicated in renal/hepatic/cardiac failure because of the increased risk of lactic acidosis.

286 (a) **True**
  (b) **False** – cf. propylthiouracil and β-blockers
  (c) **False** – Pruritus and rashes are common. They may be treated with antihistamines or propylthiouracil substitute for the carbimazole if symptoms are significant.
  (d) **True** – Methimazole, which is responsible for the therapeutic action
  (e) **True** – Potentially life-threatening/fatal

287 (a) **False**   Hypercalcemia may be a life-threatening emergency.
  (b) **False**   General management includes maintenance of hydration
  (c) **False**   with physiological saline. Plicamycin, calcitonin and
  (d) **True**   bisphosphonates reduce the plasma calcium.
  (e) **True**   Glucocorticoids reduce plasma calcium in sarcoidosis.

288 Disodium etidronate is used:

(a) Orally because it has high oral bioavailability
(b) In Paget's disease
(c) In hypercalcemia of malignancy
(d) With calcium carbonate in established vertebral osteoporosis
(e) To inhibit bone resorption and formation

289 Glucocorticoids:

(a) Reduce circulating numbers of eosinophils by inducing apoptosis
(b) Reduce circulating numbers of T lymphocytes
(c) Increase circulating numbers of neutrophils
(d) Increase circulating numbers of platelets
(e) Increase the transcription of proteins such as TNF, IL-1 and G-CSF

290 Rapid withdrawal after prolonged prednisolone administration can cause:

(a) Acute adrenal insufficiency
(b) Malaise
(c) Hypercalciuria
(d) Arthralgia
(e) Fever

291 Chronic administration of corticosteroids (iatrogenic Cushing's syndrome) results in:

(a) Increased susceptibility to opportunistic infection
(b) Hyperkalemia
(c) Hypertension
(d) Posterior capsular cataracts
(e) Proximal myopathy

292 Oral prednisolone therapy is indicated in:

(a) Fibrosing alveolitis
(b) Temporal arteritis
(c) Viral meningitis
(d) Diabetes insipidus
(e) Idiopathic thrombocytopenic purpura

288 (a) **False**   Is given intravenously or orally in spite of poor systemic
    (b) **True**   bioavailability (1–5%). It is generally well tolerated.
    (c) **True**
    (d) **True**
    (e) **True**

289 (a) **True**   Glucocorticoids reduce transcription of many
    (b) **True**   pro-inflammatory genes and induce the transcription of
    (c) **True**   others, e.g. lipocortin which inhibits phospholipase A_2 and
    (d) **True**   consequently inhibits the formation of several
                   pro-inflammatory mediators. The anti-inflammatory action
                   takes 6–8 hours to manifest after dosing.
    (e) **False** – Glucocorticosteroids inhibit the transcription of pro-
                   inflammatory cytokines such as TNF, IL-1, etc.

290 (a) **True**   Even in patients who have been successfully weaned from
    (b) **True**   chronic steroid therapy, an acute stress (e.g. trauma,
    (c) **False**   surgery, infection) may precipitate an acute adrenal crisis.
    (d) **True**
    (e) **True**

291 (a) **True** – (e.g. fungi and TB – may reactivate old tuberculous lesions)
    (b) **False** – Hypokalemia (aldosterone-like effect)
    (c) **True**
    (d) **True** – Plus local application of steroids to the eye predisposes to
                   infection
    (e) **True**

292 (a) **True** – Not curative but delays deterioriation in some patients
    (b) **True** – May prevent irreversible loss of vision
    (c) **False**
    (d) **False**
    (e) **True**

293 The risk of thromboembolic disease associated with use of the combined oral contraceptive is increased in women:

(a) Over 35 years of age
(b) Who smoke
(c) Who have been using oral contraceptives continuously for 5 years or more
(d) Who take St John's wort
(e) Who have known protein C or protein S deficiency

294 Adverse effects associated with the combined oral contraceptive include:

(a) Aggravation of asthma
(b) Stroke in women with migraine
(c) Nephrotic syndrome
(d) Peripheral neuropathy
(e) Budd–Chiari syndrome

295 The following are indications to stop the oral contraceptive immediately (pending investigation and treatment):

(a) Hemoptysis
(b) Jaundice
(c) Concurrent rifabutin therapy
(d) First (unexplained) epileptic seizure
(e) Severe unilateral calf pain

296 Bromocriptine:

(a) Stimulates lactation
(b) Is used to treat hyperprolactinemia
(c) Is a dopamine D_2-receptor agonist
(d) Commonly causes diarrhea
(e) Is effective in reducing symptoms of the syndrome of inappropriate ADH secretion

293 (a) **True**   The combined oral contraceptive should be stopped 4 weeks
    (b) **True**   before major elective surgery.
    (c) **True**
    (d) **False** – St John's wort is likely to induce metabolism of steroids
                     reducing their efficacy and side effect risks
    (e) **True** – Such patients have a high risk of thromboembolism because
                    the lack of these proteins produces a procoagulable state

294 (a) **False**   The overall acceptability of the combined pill is 80%, minor
    (b) **True**   side effects can often be controlled by a change in
    (c) **False**   preparation.
    (d) **False**
    (e) **True**

295 (a) **True**   Other indications to stop the combined oral contraceptive
    (b) **True**   immediately include sudden severe chest pain, sudden
    (c) **False**   unilateral calf pain, serious neurological effects, hepatitis,
    (d) **True**   hepatomegaly, severe depression and hypertension.
    (e) **True**

296 (a) **False** – Suppresses lactation
    (b) **True**
    (c) **True**
    (d) **False** – The commonest adverse effects are nausea and constipation
                     and orthostatic hypotension
    (e) **False** – Fluid restriction and demeclocycline is usually effective

297 Octreotide:

    (a) Is a synthetic peptide with a MW of 10 000 daltons

    (b) Is effective in reducing symptoms of carcinoid syndrome

    (c) Is effective in treating diarrhea states induced by irinotecan cancer chemotherapy

    (d) Commonly causes hyperglycemia

    (e) Is effective in the acute treatment of bleeding from esophageal varices

298 Clomiphene:

    (a) Is an estrogen receptor agonist

    (b) Is used in infertility treatment

    (c) Reduces FSH/LH secretion

    (d) Causes multiple births

    (e) Can cause acute psychotic reactions

299 Sildenafil:

    (a) Is administered by intracavernosal injection

    (b) Inhibits prostaglandin E_1

    (c) Inhibits type V phosphodiesterase

    (d) Potentiates the action of organic nitrates

    (e) May cause headaches, flushing, nasal congestion, and disturbances of color vision

297 (a) **False** – It is a synthetic octapeptide of eight amino acids MW approx. 900
    (b) **True**
    (c) **True**
    (d) **True** – It antagonizes insulin release
    (e) **True**

298 (a) **False** – It is an anti-estrogen
    (b) **True**
    (c) **False** – It blocks estrogen receptors in the hypothalamus and feedback inhibition of FSH/LH is reduced and FSH/LH secretion increase
    (d) **True**
    (e) **True**

299 (a) **False**   Sildenafil has been introduced for the treatment of
    (b) **False**   erectile dysfunction. It is taken by mouth approximately
    (c) **True**   one hour before sexual activity. Concomitant nitrates are
    (d) **True**   contraindicated.
    (e) **True**

CHAPTER EIGHT

Selective Toxicity

300 The following antibacterial drugs inhibit folic acid metabolism:

    (a) Penicillins
    (b) Monobactams
    (c) Quinolones
    (d) Trimethoprim
    (e) Sulfonamides

301 The following infections have been paired with appropriate antibacterial therapy:

    (a) Acute otitis media – amoxycillin
    (b) Acute epiglottitis in children – chloramphenicol or cefotaxime
    (c) Legionnaire's disease – erythromycin and ritampicin
    (d) Acute cystitis arising outside hospital in adults – trimethoprim
    (e) Antibiotic-associated pseudomembranous colitis – oral vancomycin

302 The following antibacterial drug combinations are of accepted benefit in the treatment of the infection cited:

    (a) Amoxycillin and cephadroxil for lower urinary tract infection in severely ill patients
    (b) Phenoxymethylpenicillin and tetracycline for acute osteomyelitis in a child under 5 years
    (c) lsoniazid, rifampicin and pyrazinamide for pulmonary TB
    (d) Erythromycin and tetracycline for septicemia
    (e) Metronidazole and nitrofurantoin for non-specific urethritis

300 (a) **False** – Inhibit cell wall synthesis
    (b) **False** – Inhibit cell wall synthesis
    (c) **False** – Inhibit DNA gyrase
    (d) **True**
    (e) **True**

301 (a) **True** – When bacterial commonly caused by group A streptococci
    (b) **True** – Caused by *H. influenzae*
    (c) **True**
    (d) **True**
    (e) **True** – Alternative oral metronidazole (NB: stop causative antibiotic)

302 (a) **False** – Intravenous gentamicin and cefuroxime
    (b) **False** – May be *Haemophilus influenzae* or *Staph. aureus* – amoxycillin and flucloxacillin is usually a satisfactory combination
    (c) **True** – Reduces the risk of resistance
    (d) **False** – Choice depends on clinical conditions, a penicillin and an aminoglycoside are a common combination in septicemia
    (e) **False** – Single agent effective (e.g. tetracycline or erythromycin)

303 The following antibacterial drugs are suitable as prophylaxis in the conditions cited:

(a) Co-amoxiclav – human and animal bites
(b) Ciprofloxacin – close adult contacts of meningococcal disease
(c) Flucloxacillin – prevention of a secondary case of diphtheria
(d) Erythromycin – whooping cough contact in an unvaccinated child under 1 year old
(e) Penicillin – traumatic CSF leakage (e.g. skull base fracture)

304 Benzylpenicillin:

(a) Is inactivated in gastric acid
(b) Is effective in streptococcal, pneumococcal and meningococcal infections
(c) Has a half-life of approximately 12 hours
(d) Is less susceptible than flucloxacillin to β-lactamase-producing strains of staphylococci
(e) Approximately 1 in 500 injections cause anaphylaxis

305 Amoxycillin:

(a) Unlike benzylpenicillin is not susceptible to β-lactamases
(b) Is effective against many strains of *H. influenzae*
(c) Is ineffective in most urinary tract infections
(d) Drug-related skin rashes may appear after dosing has stopped
(e) Drug-related skin rashes are more common in a patients with infectious mononucleosis

306 The following drugs are commonly effective in staphylococcal infections:

(a) Ampicillin
(b) Co-amoxiclav
(c) Fusidic acid
(d) Flucloxacillin
(e) Metronidazole

303 (a) **True**
   (b) **True**
   (c) **False** – Erythromycin
   (d) **True**
   (e) **True**

304 (a) **True** – Whilst phenoxymethylpenicillin (penicillin V) is stable in gastric acid and is administered orally.
   (b) **True**
   (c) **False** – Short half-life of approximately 30 minutes
   (d) **False**
   (e) **False** – 1 in 100 000

305 (a) **False**   Amoxycillin is an extended-range penicillin used for
   (b) **True**   chest infections, otitis media, urinary tract infection, biliary
   (c) **False**   infections and prevention of bacterial endocarditis. Rashes
   (d) **True**   are common and there is an especially high incidence in
   (c) **True**   infectious mononucleosis and lymphatic leukemia.

306 (a) **False** – Susceptible to β-lactamases
   (b) **True** – A combination of amoxycillin with clavulanic acid (a β-lactamase inhibitor)
   (c) **True**
   (d) **True**
   (e) **False** – Metronidazole is effective in anaerobic and protozoal infections. It is used as a part of triple therapy to eradicate *Helicobacter pylori*

307 Cefuroxime:

(a) Has activity against streptococci
(b) Has no activity against Gram-negative organisms
(c) Plasma concentrations should be monitored to avoid toxicity
(d) Is principally renally eliminated
(e) Has 10% cross-sensitivity for allergic reactions with benzylpenicillin

308 Gentamicin, an aminoglycoside:

(a) Is effective in pneumococcal pneumonia
(b) Is poorly absorbed from the gut
(c) Has an elimination half-life of approximately 12 hours if renal function is normal
(d) Cerebrospinal fluid (CSF) penetration is poor
(e) Causes irreversible eighth nerve damage

309 Chloramphenicol is usually effective in:

(a) Pulmonary tuberculosis
(b) Epiglottitis
(c) Typhoid
(d) Bacterial meningitis
(e) Bacterial conjunctivitis

310 Uses of erythromycin include:

(a) *Mycoplasma pneumoniae*
(b) Legionnaire's disease
(c) *Campylobacter* enteritis
(d) Non-specific urethritis
(e) Meningococcal meningitis

311 Erythromycin:

(a) Is poorly absorbed when given by mouth
(b) Has a shorter half-life than azithromycin
(c) The most common adverse effect is headache
(d) Inhibits cytochrome P_{450}
(e) Cannot be prescribed with amoxycillin

307 (a) **True**   Cefuroxime combines lactamase stability with activity
   (b) **False**   against streptococci, staphylococci, *H. influenzae* and *E. coli*.
   (c) **False**
   (d) **True**
   (e) **True**

308 (a) **False**   Aminoglycosides are used particularly in serious infections
   (b) **True**   such as septicemia usually in combination with a penicillin.
   (c) **False**   Blood concentration monitoring is mandatory to avoid
   (d) **True**   toxicity. The half-life is approximately 2 hours if renal
   (e) **True**   function is normal.

309 (a) **False**   Chloramphenicol has a broad spectrum and penetrates
   (b) **True**   tissues exceptionally well. Its widespread use in developing
   (c) **True**   countries has led to some resistance. Its major disadvantage
   (d) **True**   is a 1:40 000 incidence of aplastic anemia.
   (e) **True**

310 (a) **True**   Erythromycin, a macrolide, is a useful alternative to
   (b) **True**   penicillin in penicillin-allergic patients (with the notable
   (c) **True**   exception of meningitis) and is also effective against several
   (d) **True**   unusual bacteria. Clarithromycin and azithromycin are also
   (e) **False**   macrolides. They are given twice and once daily respectively
              unlike erythromycin which is given QDS. They cause fewer
              GI side effects and show better tissue penetration
              (particularly azithromycin).

311 (a) **False** – Well absorbed
   (b) **True** – Erythromycin, 1–1.5 hours; azithromycin, 40–60 hours
   (c) **False** – Gastrointestinal effects are most common
   (d) **True** – Causes accumulation of theophylline, warfarin and
              terfenadine
   (e) **False** – Often co-prescribed in community acquired pneumonia

312 Tetracyclines are used to treat:

(a) Infections caused by *Clostridium difficile*
(b) Lyme disease
(c) Acne vulgaris
(d) Systemic lupus erythematosus
(e) Non-specific urethritis

313 Metronidazole is used to treat:

(a) Trichomonal infections
(b) Amoebic dysentry
(c) Giardiasis
(d) Tetanus
(e) Gas gangrene

314 Trimethoprim:

(a) Is generally preferred to co-trimoxazole for the treatment of urinary tract infection
(b) Is generally preferred to co-trimoxazole for the treatment of pneumocystis pneumonia
(c) Should be avoided in epileptic patients
(d) Is effective treatment for Legionnaire's disease
(e) Inhibits aldehyde dehydrogenase causing a disulfiram-like reaction with alcohol

315 Ciprofloxacin:

(a) Is a drug of first choice in *Strep. pneumoniae* infections
(b) Is effective in *Pseudomonas* infections
(c) Should be avoided in children
(d) Should be avoided in epileptics
(e) Is ineffective if administered orally

316 Isoniazid:

(a) Is acetylated in the liver
(b) Is used for only the initial 2 months of the recommended 6 month anti-TB regimen in the UK
(c) Is readily absorbed from the gut
(d) Does not diffuse into the CSF
(e) Is contraindicated in children under the age of 10 years

312 (a) **False**   Oral absorption of tetracyclines is reduced by food (except
    (b) **True**   doxycycline). They must be avoided in renal impairment
    (c) **True**   (except doxycycline).
    (d) **False**
    (e) **True**

313 (a) **True**   Metronidazole has high activity against amoebae. It is widely
    (b) **True**   used prophylactically before abdominal surgery when the
    (c) **True**   rectal route is often suitable.
    (d) **False**
    (e) **True**

314 (a) **True**   Trimethoprim is generally preferred to co-trimoxazole
    (b) **False**   (trimethoprim + sulfamethoxazole) in all indications except
    (c) **False**   pneumocystis pneumonia. Hypersensitivity reactions
    (d) **False**   including Stevens–Johnson syndrome are relatively
    (e) **False**   common with sulfonamides. It is metronidazole which
                    causes a disulfiram-like reaction with alcohol.

315 (a) **False**   Oral bioavailability of the 4-fluoroquinolones is good and
    (b) **True**   they offer an oral alternative to parenteral aminoglycosides
    (c) **True**   and anti-pseudomonal penicillins for the treatment of
    (d) **True**   pseudomonal infection. Quinolones cause arthropathy in
    (e) **False**   young animals and can cause convulsions. Photosensitivity
                    also occurs.

316 (a) **True**   The standard regimen for pulmonary TB in the UK for a
    (b) **False**   UK-born patient at low risk of isoniazid resistance is
                    isoniazid, rifampicin and pyrazinamide
    (c) **True**   for 2 months followed by rifampicin and isoniazid for a
    (d) **False**   further 4 months.
    (e) **False**

317 Adverse effects associated with rifampicin include:

    (a) Hepatitis and cholestatic jaundice
    (b) Peripheral neuropathy
    (c) Convulsions
    (d) Influenza-like symptoms
    (e) Pink/red urine and tears

318 Rifampicin accelerates the hepatic metabolism of:

    (a) Corticosteroids
    (b) Warfarin
    (c) Streptomycin
    (d) Digoxin
    (e) Estrogen

319 The following adverse effects are correctly paired with a causative antituberculous drug:

    (a) Peripheral neuropathy – isoniazid
    (b) Ototoxicity – rifampicin
    (c) Hyperuricemia – pyrazinamide
    (d) Retrobulbar neuritis – ethambutol
    (e) Hepatotoxicity – streptomycin

320 Dapsone:

    (a) Is used in the treatment of amebiasis
    (b) Is indicated in multibacillary leprosy
    (c) Is used in the treatment of dermatitis herpetiformis
    (d) Is acetylated in the liver
    (e) Has cross-sensitivity with sulfonamides

321 Amphotericin B:

    (a) Is effective in local *Candida* spp. infections
    (b) Is effective in systemic *Candida* spp. infections
    (c) Is nephrotoxic
    (d) Causes hypokalemia
    (e) Is ineffective in cryptococcosis

317 (a) **True**   Serious liver damage is uncommon but minor histological
    (b) **False**   changes and rises in aminotransferase are common and in
    (c) **False**   the absence of jaundice are not an indication for stopping
    (d) **True**   treatment.
    (e) **True**

318 (a) **True**   In women using the contraceptive pill, an alternative
    (b) **True**   method of contraception should be provided. Streptomycin
    (c) **False**   and digoxin elimination is related to renal function.
    (d) **False**
    (e) **True**

319 (a) **True**   – Use prophylactic pyridoxine in diabetics, alcoholics and the
                malnourished – more common in slow acetylators
    (b) **False**   – Occurs with streptomycin
    (c) **True**   – May precipitate gout.
    (d) **True**   – Regular examinations for visual abnormalities are essential
    (e) **False**   – Occurs with isoniazid, rifampicin and pyrazinamide

320 (a) **False**   Dapsone is a sulfonamide derivative which is a competitive
    (b) **True**   inhibitor of dihydrofolate synthetase thereby blocking
    (c) **True**   dihydrofolic acid production. Clofazimine and rifampicin
    (d) **True**   are also used to treat leprosy.
    (e) **True**

321 (a) **True**   Amphotericin B is a broad spectrum antifungal although
    (b) **True**   *Aspergillus* spp. are usually resistant. It is administered
    (c) **True**   topically (lozenges), orally (suspension) or intravenously.
    (d) **True**   Intravenous lipid formulations are less toxic but more
    (e) **False**   expensive.

322 The following antifungal agents have been paired correctly with an appropriate indication:

(a) Nystatin – oral *Candida* infections
(b) Amphotericin – cryptococcal pneumonia
(c) Flucytosine – tinea pedis
(d) Clotrimazole – intertrigo
(e) Miconazole – cold sores

323 Ketoconazole:

(a) Is effective as topical and oral therapy
(b) Is active against *Aspergillus*
(c) Inhibits cortisol biosynthesis
(d) Blocks testosterone synthesis
(e) Absorption is reduced by H_2-blockers

324 Fluconazole:

(a) Oral absorption is minimal unless taken on an empty stomach
(b) Presystemic metabolism is extensive
(c) Penetrates the central nervous system well
(d) Is excreted 80% by the kidney
(e) Causes gynecomastia

325 Acyclovir (aciclovir):

(a) Inhibits viral DNA synthesis
(b) Is indicated in herpetic keratitis
(c) Should be avoided if possible in pregnancy
(d) Is indicated in herpetic meningoencephalitis
(e) Is ineffective in chicken pox

326 Foscarnet:

(a) Is indicated in cytomegalovirus (CMV) retinitis in AIDS patients
(b) Acyclovir-resistant herpes simplex virus infections
(c) Is nephrotoxic
(d) Causes fits
(e) Is usually administered by mouth or topically

322 (a) **True** – NB: bitter taste
(b) **True** – Alone or with flucytosine. Amphotericin is nephrotoxic
(c) **False** – Used with amphotericin for systemic candidosis and cryptococcosis
(d) **True** – Powder suitable
(e) **False** – Cold sores are due to herpes simplex

323 (a) **True** The systemic use of ketoconazole has waned because of the
(b) **False** high incidence of hepatic and endocrine side effects. It
(c) **True** inhibits the metabolism of cyclosporin, terfenadine and
(d) **True** astemizole.
(e) **True**

324 (a) **False** Fluconazole is a potent and broad-spectrum antifungal drug.
(b) **False** It may be used for local or systemic infections as well as
(c) **True** prophylaxis in neutropenic patients. Adverse effects are
(d) **True** gastrointestinal, erythema multiforme and hepatitis.
(e) **False**

325 (a) **True** Acyclovir is a potent and selective inhibitor of herpes
(b) **True** viruses. It may be administered as an ointment (e.g. in
(c) **True** herpetic keratitis), orally (as in shingles) or by intravenous
(d) **True** infusion as in encephalitis.
(e) **False**

326 (a) **True** Foscarnet is a nucleotide analog that inhibits DNA
(b) **True** synthesis. It is administered as an intravenous infusion in
(c) **True** both immunocompetent and immunosuppressed patients.
(d) **True**
(e) **False**

327 Adverse effects associated with the interferons include:

   (a) Hypocalcemia
   (b) Inhibition of spermatogenesis
   (c) Renal tubular acidosis
   (d) Lymphopenia
   (e) Influenza-like symptoms

328 One or more of the interferons are indicated in:

   (a) Herpes simplex encephalitis
   (b) Chronic hepatitis B infection
   (c) Chronic hepatitis C infection
   (d) Hairy cell leukemia
   (e) CMV retinitis

329 Which of the following anti-retroviral drug combinations is accepted first line therapy for patients with HIV infection?

   (a) Zidovudine (AZT) plus ddC
   (b) Zidovudine (AZT) + lamivudine + ritonavir
   (c) Ritonavir + amprenavir
   (d) Zidovudine (AZT) + lamivudine + nevirapine
   (e) Zidovudine (AZT) + stavudine (d4T) + nevirapine

330 Properties of HIV protease inhibitors include:

   (a) Cause hypertrigyceridemia and truncal fat redistribution
   (b) Are most effective of the anti-retrovirals at reducing number of plasma HIV RNA copies
   (c) Oral bioavailability is consistent and >95%
   (d) Cause many drug–drug interactions due to inhibition of CYP3A
   (e) HIV resistance to one agent in the class usually means cross-resistance to others

331 The following are used to treat *Pneumocystis carinii* pneumonia (PCP) in patients with HIV infection:

   (a) Aztreonam
   (b) Intravenous co-trimoxazole
   (c) Ciprofloxacin
   (d) Pentamidine
   (e) Glucocorticoids if the arterial Po_2 is less than 60 mmHg

327 (a) **False** – Associated with foscarnet
(b) **False** – Associated with ganciclovir which is indicated in severe CMV infection in immunocompromised patients
(c) **False** – Associated with amphotericin
(d) **True**
(e) **True**

328 (a) **False**   Interferons are glycoproteins secreted by cells infected with
(b) **True**   viruses or foreign double-stranded DNA. They are non-
(c) **True**   antigenic and species specific. α-Interferon is combined
(d) **True**   with ribavirin for the treatment of hepatitis C.
(e) **False**   β-Interferon is licensed for the treatment of multiple sclerosis.

329 (a) **False**   Triple therapy: two nucleoside analogs + inhibitor or + non-
(b) **True**   nucleoside reverse transcriptase inhibitor is accepted first
(c) **False**   line. See *TCP*, Chapter 45, p. 523.
(d) **True**
(e) **False**   AZT + d4T antagonistic *in vitro* at least. Not used clinically

330 (a) **True**   Saquinavir, retinovir, indinavir and nelfinavir are anti-HIV
(b) **True**   protease inhibitors
(c) **False**
(d) **True**
(e) **True**

331 (a) **False**   High dose co-trimoxazole is first line standard treatment
(b) **True**   for PCP in patients with HIV infection. After recovery,
(c) **False**   secondary prophylaxis with oral co-trimoxazole is usual.
(d) **True**
(e) **True**

332 Chloroquine:

(a) Only injures *Plasmodium* when the parasite is extracellular
(b) Must be given by intravenous infusion in *P. vivax* malaria
(c) Can cause irreversible visual loss when used as prolonged therapy
(d) Should not be co-prescribed with proguanil
(e) Is contraindicated in children under 10 years

333 The following acute *Plasmodium* infections are paired with their appropriate treatment:

(a) Falciparurn malaria in West Africa – quinine
(b) Cerebral malaria in West Africa – quinine and chloroquine
(c) *P. vivax* – chloroquine followed by primaquine
(d) *P. vivax* in a pregnant woman – chloroquine, the primaquine being postponed until after delivery
(e) Falciparum malaria in East Africa in a pregnant woman – halofantrine

334 Quinine sulfate:

(a) Is the drug of choice in chloroquine-resistant falciparum malaria
(b) Is available for intravenous and oral use
(c) Is effective in eradicating the hepatic parasites in *P. vivax* malaria
(d) Is contraindicated in renal failure
(e) Large therapeutic doses cause tinnitus

335 The following adverse effects are paired with a causative antimalarial drug:

(a) Lichenoid skin eruption – chloroquine
(b) Stevens–Johnson syndrome – quinine
(c) Hallucinations – mefloquine
(d) Prolongation of QTc – proguanil
(e) Hemolytic anemia – primaquine

332 (a) **False**   Chloroquine is one of the most widely used antimalarial
   (b) **False**   drugs. Unfortunately the incidence of falciparum resistance
   (c) **True**   to chloroquine is becoming more widespread.
   (d) **False**
   (e) **False**

333 (a) **True**
   (b) **False** – Quinine and chloroquine are antagonistic
   (c) **True** – Primaquine is required to destroy the parasites in the liver
      and prevent relapse
   (d) **True** – After the standard course of chloroquine as for a
      non-pregnant patient, chloroquine is continued weekly
      until delivery
   (e) **False** – Falciparum malaria is particularly dangerous in the last
      trimester – use quinine

334 (a) **True** – If resistance is not a possibility, chloroquine may be used
   (b) **True**
   (c) **False** – Primaquine
   (d) **False**
   (e) **True** – Cinchonism, which also includes deafness, headache,
      nausea and visual disturbance

335 (a) **True** – Other choroquine side effects include convulsions, visual
      disturbances, depigmentation, hair loss and it is very toxic
      in overdose
   (b) **False** – Recognized with pyrimethamine with sulfadoxine
      (Fansidar®)
   (c) **True** – Also potentiates the bradycardic effect of β-blockers
   (d) **False**
   (e) **True** – In glucose 6-phosphate dehydrogenase deficient patients

336 The following infections have been paired with appropriate drug therapy:

(a) *Trypanosoma gambiense* (African sleeping sickness), early stages – pentamidine and suramin
(b) Giardiasis – metronidazole
(c) *Taenia saginata* (a tapeworm) – emetine
(d) Threadworm – mebendazole
(e) *Toxocara canis* – pyrantel

337 The following cytotoxic drugs are extremely emetogenic:

(a) Cyclophosphamide
(b) Methotrexate
(c) 5-Fluorouracil
(d) Mustine
(e) Cisplatin

338 The following cytotoxic drugs may be associated with prolonged myelosuppression:

(a) Chlorambucil
(b) Melphalan
(c) BCNU (1,3-bis (2 chloroethyl-l-nitrourea))
(d) Bleomycin
(e) Vincristine

339 During cancer chemotherapy:

(a) Infection is the commonest life-threatening complication
(b) Infection is often acquired from the patient's own gut flora
(c) If infection occurs, pyrexia is usually absent
(d) Men and women must be strongly advised to avoid conception
(e) There is a danger of inducing second malignancies

340 Cyclophosphamide:

(a) Is normally used in combination with other cytotoxic agents
(b) Is an alkylating agent
(c) Causes granulocytopenia
(d) Causes nausea and vomiting
(e) Causes alopecia

336 (a) **True**
   (b) **True**
   (c) **False** – A single dose of praziquantel is curative
   (d) **True** – Pyrantel also effective
   (e) **False** – Diethylcarbamazine, corticosteroids may be needed to treat allergic reactions to dying larvae

337 (a) **True**   Nausea and vomiting are often the principal immediate
   (b) **False**   toxic effects associated with cytotoxic chemotherapy. To
   (c) **False**   avoid tissue necrosis, another immediate effect, expert
   (d) **True**   attention to vascular access is mandatory.
   (e) **True**

338 (a) **True**   There are two patterns of bone marrow recovery after
   (b) **True**   suppression (*TCP*, Fig 47.4), rapid and delayed. Vincristine
   (c) **True**   and bleomycin seldom cause myelosuppression. Vincristine
   (d) **False**   is associated with peripheral or autonomic neuropathy. It is
   (e) **False**   very irritant and must never be given into the intrathecal space. Extravasation from a vein causes profound local ulceration.

339 (a) **True**   Broad-spectrum antibacterial treatment must be started
   (b) **True**   empirically in febrile neutropenic patients without waiting
   (c) **False**   for culture results. The effect on fertility and the risk of
   (d) **True**   future fetal abnormalities are very variable. Alkylating
   (e) **True**   agents are particularly harmful. Successful pregnancies are not unusual in women at least 6 months after completion of chemotherapy. Sperm storage should be considered.

340 (a) **True**   Cyclophosphamide is most useful in the treatment of
   (b) **True**   various lymphomas and leukemias and in myeloma but it
   (c) **True**   also has some effect in other malignancies (e.g. breast
   (d) **True**   cancer, small cell lung cancer). It may be given by mouth or
   (e) **True**   intravenous injection.

341 Sterile hemorrhagic cystitis is associated with:

    (a) Cyclophosphamide
    (b) Ifosfamide
    (c) Acrolein
    (d) Corticosteroids
    (e) Mesna

342 Methotrexate:

    (a) Is a folinic acid antagonist
    (b) The toxicity of high doses can be reduced by giving folinic acid 24 hours after the methotrexate
    (c) Doses should be reduced if allopurinol is administered
    (d) Chronic treatment can cause cirrhosis
    (e) Is the treatment of choice for choriocarcinoma

343 The following cytotoxic drugs are paired with a characteristic adverse effect:

    (a) Doxorubicin – peripheral neuropathy
    (b) Etoposide – alopecia
    (c) Daunorubicin – cardiomyopathy
    (d) Methotrexate – oral ulceration
    (e) 6-Mercaptopurine – pulmonary fibrosis

344 During cisplatin therapy:

    (a) Pretreatment hydration is mandatory
    (b) Pretreatment with ondansetron reduces the nausea and vomiting
    (c) Visual disturbances are common
    (d) Magnesium supplements are usually given
    (e) Nephrotoxicity is dose related and dose limiting

345 Recombinant human erythropoietin is used to treat:

    (a) Iron deficient anemia when iron is malabsorbed
    (b) Pernicious anemia
    (c) Anemia of chronic renal failure
    (d) AZT-induced anemia
    (e) Clozapine-induced agranulocytosis

341 (a) **True** Mesna protects the urinary tract against the irritant
    (b) **True** metabolites of cyclophosphamide and ifosfamide and in
    (c) **True** particular acrolein, a metabolite of these agents.
    (d) **False**
    (e) **False**

342 (a) **True**
    (b) **True**
    (c) **False** – Allopurinol antagonizes methotrexate by increasing purine
           availability
    (d) **True**
    (e) **True**

343 (a) **False** – Peripheral neuropathy is common with vincristine
    (b) **True** – Etoposide is particularly active in small cell lung cancer
    (c) **True**
    (d) **True**
    (e) **False** – Pulmonary fibrosis is associated with busulfan therapy

344 (a) **True** Cisplatin is of value in metastatic germ cell cancers
    (b) **True** (seminoma and teratoma). Carboplatin is widely used in
    (c) **False** advanced ovarian cancer and lung cancer (especially in
    (d) **True** small cell lung cancer). It is generally better tolerated than
    (e) **True** cisplatin; however it is more myelosuppressive. Oxaliplatin
               is used in metastatic colorectal cancer in combination with
               fluorouracil and folinic acid. Neurotoxicity is dose limiting.

345 (a) **False** – Use parenteral iron
    (b) **False** – Use parenteral vitamin B_{12}
    (c) **True**
    (d) **True**
    (e) **False**

346 Filgrastim (human granulocyte colony stimulating factor):

(a) Is usually administered by subcutaneous injection
(b) Causes immediate transient neutropenia
(c) Is used in myeloid leukemia
(d) Stimulates proliferation and differentiation of progenitor cells of all granulocyte lines
(e) Causes bone pain

346 (a) **True** – Often self-administered
    (b) **True**
    (c) **False** – Increases proliferation of the malignant clone
    (d) **True**
    (e) **True** – Also myalgia, fever, splenomegaly, thrombocytopenia and
                 abnormal liver enzymes

CHAPTER NINE

Clinical Immunopharmacology

347 Azathioprine:

- (a) Is metabolized to 6-mercaptopurine
- (b) Inhibits delayed hypersensitivity (cell mediated immunity) and those aspects of inflammation that require cell division
- (c) Is administered by subcutaneous injection
- (d) Causes hemopoietic suppression
- (e) Concurrent allopurinol increases the clearance of azathioprine

348 Cyclophosphamide is used as an immunosuppressive in the following diseases:

- (a) Cystic fibrosis
- (b) Autoimmune thrombocytopenia (ITP)
- (c) Nephrotic syndrome with minimal microscopic glomerular changes
- (d) Nephritis due to systemic lupus erythematosus
- (e) Wegener's granulomatosis

349 Glucocorticoids inhibit:

- (a) Platelet thromboxane A_2 synthesis
- (b) Histamine release
- (c) Leukotriene C_4 and D_4 synthesis
- (d) Lipocortin synthesis
- (e) Neutrophil production

350 The following agents are used to prevent or treat graft-versus-host disease:

- (a) Glucocorticosteroids
- (b) Cyclosporin
- (c) Mycophenolate mofetil
- (d) Tacrolimus
- (e) Basiliximab

347 (a) **True**   Azathioprine is an antimetabolite and thus most
    (b) **True**   effective on proliferating cells. It is administered by mouth
    (c) **False**   and metabolized to its active moiety – 6 mercaptopurine.
    (d) **True**   It is used as an adjunct to prevent transplant rejection and
    (e) **False**   also in the treatment of autoimmune diseases such as
                  systemic lupus erythematosus and chronic active hepatitis.
                  Owing to its potential toxicity (bone marrow) it is usually
                  reserved for situations in which corticosteroids alone are
                  inadequate.

348 (a) **False**   Cyclophosphamide, in addition to its uses in oncology as a
    (b) **False**   cytotoxic drug, is particularly valuable in aggressive
    (c) **True**   auto-immune diseases inhibiting lymphocyte proliferation.
    (d) **True**
    (e) **True**

349 (a) **False**   Glucocorticoids reduce the transcription of pro-
    (b) **True**   inflammatory mediators and inhibit type I, II, III and IV
    (c) **True**   hypersensitivity reactions. They are the most widely used
    (d) **False**   immunosuppressive agents. They inhibit eicosanoid
    (e) **False**   synthesis in nucleated cells by increasing the production of
                  lipocortin, an inhibitor of PLA_2, and increase the
                  neutrophil count in peripheral blood.

350 (a) **True**
    (b) **True**   – Specific T lymphocyte suppressor, primarily against
                 T helper cells
    (c) **True**   – Need regular blood counts.
    (d) **True**   – Is neurotoxic and nephrotoxic
    (e) **True**   – Monoclonal antibody that prevents T cell proliferation

351 Adverse effects associated with ciclosporin include:

    (a) Nephrotoxicity
    (b) Nausea and gastrointestinal disturbances
    (c) Alopecia
    (d) Tremor
    (e) Hypokalemia

352 Administration of basiliximab (IL-2 receptor blocking antibody) may cause the following side effects:

    (a) Anaphylactic shock
    (b) Delayed symptoms of severe dyspnea and wheeze
    (c) Fever and chills
    (d) Aseptic meningitis
    (e) Cardiomyopathy

353 Mycophenolate mofetil:

    (a) Is a prodrug
    (b) Inhibits inosine monophosphate dehydrogenase, impairing *de novo* purine synthesis in T and B cells
    (c) Is given intravenously
    (d) Causes leukopenia
    (e) Is used as adjunct therapy in solid organ transplantation and is more effective than azathioprine

354 The following agents inhibit the metabolism of ciclosporin:

    (a) Diltiazem
    (b) Ketoconazole
    (c) Cimetidine
    (d) Rifampicin
    (e) Vancomycin

355 The following are indicated in the management of acute anaphylactic shock following a bee sting out of hospital and without monitoring facilities:

    (a) Intramuscular adrenaline (epinephrine) (0.5–1 mL, 1 in 1000)
    (b) Intravenous adrenaline (epinephrine) (10 mL, 1 in 10 000)
    (c) Intravenous hydrocortisone
    (d) Intravenous chlorpheniramine
    (e) Oxygen

351 (a) **True** – Also may cause hypertension. Nephrotoxicity may be
reduced by concurrent calcium channel blockade
   (b) **True** – In up to 20% of patients
   (c) **False** – Hirsutism
   (d) **True** – May be an early sign of toxic plasma concentrations
   (e) **False** – Causes hyperkalemia

352 (a) **True** – Any murine/humanized monoclonal antibody when given
to man may cause anaphylaxis
   (b) **True** – Manifestation of a delayed hypersensitivity reactions
   (c) **True**
   (d) **False** – Intravenous human normal immunoglobulin (HNIG) in
high dose can cause this
   (e) **False**

353 (a) **True**   It is an ester of mycophenolic acid, the latter undergoes
   (b) **True**   hepatic glucuronidation to an inactive metabolite. Blocks
   (c) **False**   purine synthesis in proliferating lymphocytes and may
   (d) **True**   reduce production of pro-inflammatory cytokines. Is given
   (e) **True**   orally. Antacids decrease its absorption. Also causes
   gastrointestinal side effects.

354 (a) **True** – CYP3A4 inhibitors block cyclosporin (and tacrolimus)
metabolism increasing the risk of toxicity if the dose of
immunosuppressant is not reduced
   (b) **True**
   (c) **True**
   (d) **False** – Rifampicin (and all rifamycins) induce CYP3A4 reducing
ciclosporin blood concentrations for the same dose
   (e) **False** – Vancomycin may however potentiate the nephrotoxicity of
ciclosporin.

355 (a) **True** – Life saving
   (b) **False** – May induce ventricular fibrillation
   (c) **True** – But takes 4–6 hours to be of benefit
   (d) **True**
   (e) **True** – If hypotensive intravenous fluids may also be of value and
may be available in an ambulance.

356 Fexofenadine:

    (a) Is a H_1-receptor antagonist
    (b) Is used as a sedative in children
    (c) Is an effective antiemetic
    (d) Is used prophylactically in hayfever
    (e) Plasma concentrations when very high can lead to prolonged QTc and torsades de pointes

357 The following are successfully used in the management of allergic rhinitis (hayfever):

    (a) Oral H_3 receptor antagonists
    (b) Desensitization with a mix of grass pollen, cat dander and house dust mite
    (c) Nasal cromoglycate
    (d) Nasal salbutamol
    (e) Nasal glucocorticosteroids

358 Most children would have received the following vaccines before entry into primary school:

    (a) Measles, mumps and rubella
    (b) Influenza
    (c) Diphtheria, tetanus and pertussis
    (d) Polio
    (e) Smallpox

356 (a) **False**   Fexofenadine, terfenadine, astemizole, cetirizine and
(b) **False**   loratadine are "non-sedative" antihistamines.
(c) **False**
(d) **True**
(e) **False** – Fexofenadine is the non-cardiotoxic metabolite of
terfenadine

357 (a) **False**   Avoidance of allergens is ideal but rarely practical. With the
(b) **False**   exception of oral H_1-blockers, local therapy is preferred.
(c) **True**   If indicated desensitization therapy with a single allergen is
(d) **False**   acceptable, but the risk of anaphylaxis is high and it should
(e) **True**   only be undertaken in specialist allergy clinics.

358 (a) **True**   Live vaccines should be avoided in the immunosuppressed.
(b) **False**   Meningococcal group C conjugate vaccine provides
(c) **True**   protection against serogroup C of *N. meningitidis* and is now
(d) **True**   part of the primary course of childhood immunization.
(e) **False**   Meningococcal polysaccharide A and C vaccine is
recommended for those traveling to certain areas during
epidemics. *Haemophilus influenzae* b vaccine is administered
during the second year of life.

CHAPTER TEN

The Skin and the Eye

359 Acne vulgaris:

  (a) Can be effectively treated with topical retinoic acid
  (b) May be precipitated by oral methylprednisolone
  (c) Is caused by propionibacteria
  (d) Cold tar treatment reduces the severity of lesions
  (e) Can be exacerbated by oral acyclovir

360 Isotretinoin:

  (a) Is a synthetic vitamin D analog
  (b) The usual course of treatment is 2 weeks
  (c) Is teratogenic
  (d) Causes hirsutism
  (e) Is eliminated from the body over a period of weeks

361 The following are effective in the management of eczema:

  (a) Topical betamethasone
  (b) Topical α-tocopherol
  (c) Dithranol
  (d) Calcipotriol
  (e) Emulsifying ointment

362 Local application of the following are of benefit in the management of psoriasis:

  (a) Acitretin
  (b) Salicylic acid
  (c) Psoralens
  (d) Dithranol
  (e) Calcipotriol

359 (a) **True**   Acne vulgaris occurs in at least 90% of adolescents. The
    (b) **True**   topical use of peeling agents such as benzoyl peroxide or
    (c) **True**   retinoic acid on a regular basis is usually all that is
    (d) **False**   necessary. In more severe cases oral antibacterial drugs are
    (e) **False**   beneficial and if this is ineffective oral isotretinoin may be
                    considered by specialists.

360 (a) **False**   Isotretinoin is a vitamin A analog it is prescribed under
    (b) **False**   hospital supervision usually for 4 months.
    (c) **True** – There is a persistent risk of teratogenicity for at least 1
                    month after stopping oral therapy
    (d) **False**
    (e) **True**

361 (a) **True**   If the eczema is wet the topical use of drying agents such as
    (b) **False**   lotions of aluminum acetate or calamine are useful. When
    (c) **False**   the lesions are dry and scaly the use of moisturizing cream
    (d) **False**   (e.g. E45) combined with a keratolytic is beneficial. Topical
    (e) **True**   corticosteroids are often required. Nocturnal pruritus may
                    be relieved by sedative antihistamines.

362 (a) **False** – Acitretin is an oral retinoid used in severe, resistant or
                    complicated psoriasis
    (b) **True** – Enhances rate of loss of surface scale
    (c) **False** – PUVA (photochemotherapy using an oral psoralen with
                    long wave ultraviolet radiation) is an effective but
                    unlicensed treatment for psoriasis
    (d) **True** – Irritates normal skin
    (e) **True** – Does not irritate normal skin

363 The following drugs are recognized causes of Stevens–Johnson syndrome:

(a) Co-trimoxazole
(b) Amoxicillin
(c) L-Thyroxine
(d) Phenytoin
(e) Lamotrigine

364 The following infections/infestations are paired with their appropriate treatment:

(a) *Candida vulvovaginitis* – topical ketoconazole
(b) Fungal nail infections – oral griseofulvin
(c) Tinea corporis – topical clotrimazole
(d) Initial or recurrent genital herpes simplex – oral aciclovir (acyclovir)
(e) Scabies – topical malathion

365 Adminstration of the following eye drops/ ointments can produce the correctly paired systemic effects :

(a) Carteolol – bradycardia
(b) Acyclovir – alopecia
(c) Gentamicin – renal tubular necrosis
(d) Prednisolone – hypercalcemia
(e) Pilocarpine – dry mouth

366 Dilatation of the pupil (mydriasis) is produced by:

(a) Cyclopentolate
(b) Dorzolamide
(c) Atropine
(d) Phenylephrine
(e) Ketorolac

367 In the treatment of open angle glaucoma the following drugs are effective:

(a) Acetozolamide
(b) Chlorpheniramine
(c) Dexamethasone
(d) Latanoprost
(e) Timolol

363 (a) **True**   All sulfonamides and β-lactam antibacterials can cause this problem.
    (b) **True**
    (c) **False**
    (d) **True**
    (e) **True**

364 (a) **True**   With unusual/recurrent skin infections consider diabetes
    (b) **True**   mellitus or immunosuppression.
    (c) **True**
    (d) **True**
    (e) **True**

365 (a) **True** – Intraocular administered doses avoid hepatic first pass metabolism and can lead to bradycardia
    (b) **False**
    (c) **False** – Not enough absorbed to cause systemic toxicity
    (d) **False**
    (e) **True** – With high doses enough can be absorbed to produce systemic anticholinergic effects.

366 (a) **True** – Muscarinic (M3 in the eye) receptor antagonist blocks action of sphincter muscle of the iris
    (b) **False** – Topical carbonic anhydrase inhibitor
    (c) **True** – Muscarinic (M3 in the eye) receptor antagonist blocks action of sphincter muscle of the iris
    (d) **True** – Stimulates α_1-adrenoreceptors constricting the radial muscle of the iris
    (e) **False** – Is a topical and systemic NSAID

367 (a) **True** – Carbonic anhydrase inhibitor given systemically reduces production of the aqueous humor
    (b) **False** – First generation antihistamine will dilate the pupil (due to its anticholinergic properties) worsening glaucoma
    (c) **False** – Steroids can exacerbate glaucoma in certain genetically predisposed patients
    (d) **True** – $PGF_{2\alpha}$ analogue lowers intraocular pressure by increasing uveoscleral flow
    (e) **True** – β-Adrenergic antagonist reduces secretion/formation of aqueous humor

CHAPTER ELEVEN

Clinical Toxicology

368 Methadone:

    (a) Has the potential to cause dependence
    (b) Can only be prescribed to registered addicts by doctors with a special license
    (c) Is usually administered as an elixir
    (d) Depresses the cough center
    (e) Effects are reversed by naloxone

369 The following are clinical signs consistent with heroin (diamorphine) intoxication:

    (a) Hypertension
    (b) Rapid respiratory rate
    (c) Hypothermia
    (d) Pin-point pupils
    (e) Slurred speech

370 Features of the opioid withdrawal syndrome include:

    (a) Yawning
    (b) Rhinorrhea
    (c) Mydriasis
    (d) Diarrhea
    (e) Tremor

371 Specific causes of death which are positively related to smoking include:

    (a) Ischemic heart disease
    (b) Cancer of the esophagus
    (c) Emphysema
    (d) Aortic aneurysm
    (e) Cancer of the tongue

368 (a) **True** Methadone elixir/mixture is the mainstay of many drug
   (b) **False** addiction clinics. It has a long half-life of 15–55 hours and
   (c) **True** it is very difficult to administer these oral formulations as
   (d) **True** an injection.
   (e) **True**

369 (a) **False** Initially intravenous heroin produces an intense euphoria
   (b) **False** for several seconds (often accompanied by
   (c) **True** nausea/vomiting). Many chronic users often claim the only
   (d) **True** effect is remission from abstinence symptoms.
   (e) **True**

370 (a) **True** Withdrawal symptoms generally start at the time the next
   (b) **True** dose would usually be given and their intensity is related to
   (c) **True** the usual dose. For heroin, symptoms usually reach a
   (d) **True** maximum at 36–72 hours and gradually subside over the
   (e) **True** next 5–10 days. Lofexidine, an α_2-antagonist, alleviates
                many of the withdrawal symptoms. Loperamide helps
                reduce the diarrhea.

371 (a) **True** In the UK, in men under 70 years, the ratio of death rate
   (b) **True** among cigarette smokers to non-smokers is 2:1. To assist
   (c) **True** smokers to give up, nicotine chewing gum, patches,
   (d) **True** sublingual tablets and spray are available.
   (e) **True** Afebutamone/bupropion has also been introduced as a
                adjunct to smoking cessation. It may impair performance
                of skilled tasks such as driving.

372 There is an increased rate of metabolism of the following drugs in smokers:

(a) Diazepam
(b) Phenytoin
(c) Ethanol
(d) Warfarin
(e) Theophylline

373 Ethyl alcohol (ethanol):

(a) The majority of oral ethanol is absorbed from the small intestine
(b) Ethanol delays gastic emptying
(c) 95% of ingested ethanol is metabolized
(d) Ethanol elimination demonstrates first order kinetics
(e) Is second to heroin as the most important drug of dependence in Western Europe

374 Cardiovascular complications associated with alcohol consumption include:

(a) Atrial fibrillation
(b) Buerger's disease
(c) Cardiomyopathy
(d) Coronary artery disease
(e) Peripheral vascular disease

375 Delirium tremens:

(a) Occurs in approximately 60% of patients withdrawing from alcohol
(b) Has a mortality of 5–10%
(c) Benzodiazepines are contraindicated
(d) Thiamine should be administered parenterally
(e) Phenytoin should be administered prophylactically to prevent convulsions

376 Chronic use of anabolic steroids is associated with:

(a) Pancreatitis
(b) Ototoxicity
(c) Hepatic tumors
(d) Cardiomyopathy
(e) Peripheral neuropathy

372 (a) **False**   In addition to pharmacokinetic differences, smokers may
     (b) **False**   exhibit altered pharmacodynamic responses (e.g. smokers
     (c) **False**   show less CNS depression after a standard dose of
     (d) **False**   diazepam than non-smokers).
     (e) **True**

373 (a) **True**   It has been estimated that the incidence of alcoholism in
     (b) **True**   North America and Western Europe is nearly 5% of the
     (c) **True**   population. Ethanol is a weak inducer of its own
     (d) **False**   metabolism but is a more potent inducer of the
     (e) **False**   metabolism of drugs whose principal metabolic process is
                via CYP_{450} particularly CYP_{4502EI} and differences in rate of
                ethanol metabolism are principally genetic.

374 (a) **True**
     (b) **False** – Associated with smoking
     (c) **True**
     (d) **False** – Associated with smoking
     (e) **False** – Associated with smoking

375 (a) **False** – < 10%
     (b) **True**
     (c) **False** – Chlormethiazole and benzodiazepines (long half-life) are
                     suitable sedatives
     (d) **True** – To avoid precipitation of acute thiamine deficiency when
                    intravenous dextrose/oral carbohydrates are administered
     (e) **False**

376 (a) **False**   Anabolic steroids are abused by athletes to build up muscle
     (b) **False**   tissue.
     (c) **True**
     (d) **True**
     (e) **False**

377 Methylenedioxymethylamphetamine (MDMA or ecstasy):

(a) Has agonist properties at the 5HT$_2$ receptor
(b) Has mixed hallucinogenic and stimulant properties
(c) Occasionally causes hyperplexia
(d) In chronic use has been associated with increased impulsivity and impaired memory
(e) Chronic usage may cause irreversible degeneration of serotonergic nerves

378 The combination of coma, dilated pupils, hyperreflexia and tachycardia is consistent with overdose of the following drugs when taken alone:

(a) Co-proxamol
(b) Dothiepin
(c) Aspirin
(d) Amitriptyline
(e) Lorazepam

377 (a) **True**   MDMA is widely abused for its stimulant and
    (b) **True**   hallucinogenic properties. It is metabolized by CYP 2D6
    (c) **True**   which it inhibits for up to 2 weeks following a single dose.
    (d) **True**   It is occasionally associated with hyperpyrexia,
    (e) **True**   hyponatremia, rhabdomyolysis and coma.

378 (a) **False**   A meticulous, rapid but thorough clinical examination is
    (b) **True**   essential not only to exclude other causes of coma or
    (c) **False**   behavior, but also because the symptoms and signs may
    (d) **True**   be characteristic of certain poisons.
    (e) **False**

Table 4 Clinical manifestations of some common poisons

Symptoms/signs of acute overdose	Common poisons
Coma, hypotension, flaccidity	Benzodiazepines and other hypnosedatives, alcohol
Coma, pin-point pupils, hypoventilation	Opioids
Coma, dilated pupils, hyperreflexia, tachycardi(a)	Tricyclic antidepressants, phenothiazines; other drugs with anticholinergic properties
Restlessness, hypertonia, hyperreflexia, pyrexia	Amphetamines, MDMA, anticholinergic agents
Convulsions	Tricyclic antidepressants, phenothiazines, carbon monoxide, monoamine oxidase inhibitors, mefenamic acid, theophylline, hypoglycemic agents, lithium, cyanide
Tinnitus, overbreathing, pyrexia, sweating, flushing, usually alert	Salicylates
Burns in mouth, dysphagia, abdominal pain	Corrosives, caustics, paraquat

379 The following suspected overdoses are indications for emergency measurement of drug concentration:

(a) Iron
(b) Methanol
(c) Amitriptyline
(d) Temazepam
(e) Salicylates

380 Alkaline diuresis enhances the elimination of:

(a) Amphetamine
(b) Salicylates
(c) Theophylline
(d) Phenobarbitone
(e) Dothiepin

379 (a) **True**
(b) **True**
(c) **False**
(d) **False**
(e) **True**

Table 5 Common indications for emergency measurements of drug concentration

Suspected overdose	Effect on management
Paracetamol	Administration of antidotes – acetylcysteine or methionine
Iron	Administration of antidote – desferrioxamine
Methanol/ethylene glycol	Administration of antidote – ethanol ± dialysis
Lithium	Dialysis
Salicylates	Simple rehydration or alkaline diuresis or dialysis
Theophylline	Necessity of ITU admission

380 (a) **False**   Methods to increase poison elimination are appropriate in
(b) **True**   less than 5% of overdose causes.
(c) **False**
(d) **True**
(e) **False**

Table 6 Methods and indications for enhancement of poison elimination

Method(s)	Poison
Alkaline diuresis	Salicylates, phenobarbitone
Acid diuresis	Phencyclidine, ?amphetamine
Hemodialysis (peritoneal dialysis is also effective but two to three times less efficient)	Salicylates, methanol, ethylene glycol, lithium, phenobarbitone
Charcoal hemoperfusion (rarely necessary)	Barbiturates, theophylline disopyramide
"Gastrointestinal dialysis" using activated charcoal	Salicylates, most anticonvulsants, digoxin, theophylline, quinine

381 The following poisons/drugs have been correctly paired with an appropriate antidote/specific measure:

(a) Paracetamol – acetylcysteine
(b) Iron – desferrioxamine
(c) Dextropropoxyphene – naloxone
(d) Organophosphorus insecticides – dicobalt edatate
(e) Methanol – ethanol

381 (a) **True**
    (b) **True**
    (c) **True**
    (d) **False**
    (e) **True**

Table 7 Antidotes and other specific measures

Overdose drug	Antidote/other specific measures
Paracetamol	Acetylcysteine i.v.
	Methionine p$^{\circ}$.
Iron	Desferrioxamine
Cyanide	Oxygen, amyl nitrate (inhalation), dicobalt edetate i.v., sodium nitrate i.v., followed by sodium thiosulfate i.v.
Benzodiazepines	Flumazenil i.v.
β-Blocker	Glucagon
	Atropine
	Isoprenaline
Carbon monoxide	Oxygen
	Hyperbaric oxygen
Methanol/ethylene glycol	Ethanol fomepizole
Lead	Sodium calcium edetate i.v.
	Penicillamine p$^{\circ}$.
	Dimercaptosuccinic acid (DMSA) i.v. or p$^{\circ}$.
Mercury	Dimercaptopropane suifonate (DMPS)
	Dimercaptosuccinic acid (DMSA)
	Dimercaprol
	Penicillamine
Opioids	Naloxone
Organophosphorus insecticides	Atropine, pralidoxime
Digoxin	Digoxin specific fab antibody fragments
Calcium channel blockers	Calcium chloride or gluconate i.v. glucagon
Insulin	50% dextrose i.v.
	glucagon i.v. or i.m.

*NB: DMSSA and DMPS are not licensed in the UK. Advice should be sought from a Poisons Information Centre.

382 An 18-year-old woman is admitted 2 hours after taking 50 paracetamol and 50 aspirin tablets. The following statements are correct:

(a) She is likely to be in a grade IV coma
(b) Stomach washout is indicated
(c) Acetylcysteine should be administered
(d) Blood gases are likely to show a mixed metabolic acidosis/respiratory alkalosis
(e) If the prothrombin time is prolonged acetylcysteine is contraindicated

383 The following are confirmed aphrodisiacs:

(a) Ginseng
(b) Oysters
(c) Extract of rhino horn
(d) Passion fruit
(e) Vitamin E

382 (a) **False**   Paracetamol and salicylate overdoses only very rarely
   (b) **True**   cause coma acutely. Salicylate overdose is an indication
   (c) **True**   for late stomach washout (some authorities disagree).
   (d) **True**   Acetylcysteine is a potentially life-saving antidote in
   (e) **False**   paracetamol overdose.

383 (a) **False**   The authors recommend champagne!
   (b) **False**
   (c) **False**
   (d) **False**
   (e) **False**

CHAPTER TWELVE

Practice MCQ Examination

Mark +2 for a correct response, 0 for no response and –1 for an incorrect response. 50% is the pass mark for the examination (i.e. 300/600 score marks). Allow 90 minutes in one sitting to complete this mock examination.

1 The following receptors have been paired correctly with their agonist:

(a) β_1-receptor – esmolol
(b) β_2-receptor – salmeterol
(c) α_1-receptor – noradrenaline
(d) 5-HT$_{1D}$ receptor – sumatriptan
(e) Dopamine D$_2$-receptor – risperidone

2 The following decrease the rate of gastric emptying and hence the rate of oral drug absorption:

(a) Chlorpheniramine
(b) Domperidone
(c) Paracetamol (acetaminophen)
(d) Migraine
(e) Metoclopramide

3 A "healthy" 75-year-old man will eliminate the following drugs more slowly than a "healthy" 25-year-old man:

(a) Gentamicin
(b) Digoxin
(c) Dalteparin
(d) Atenolol
(e) Ethambutol

1 (a) **False** – Esmolol is a β_1 selective receptor antagonist with a very short duration of action
  (b) **True**
  (c) **True**
  (d) **True** – Sumatriptan is used to treat migraine
  (e) **False** – Most antipsychotic drugs are D_2-antagonists. Risperidone is an "atypical" antipsychotic drug which blocks D_2-receptors but blocks $5HT_2$ receptors in particular

2 (a) **True** – Anticholinergic action
  (b) **False** – Motility stimulant. Domperidone does not readily cross the blood–brain barrier and is much less likely to cause dystonic reactions than metoclopramide
  (c) **False**
  (d) **True** – Hence the rationale for combining metoclopramide with minor analgesics in migraine
  (e) **False** – Motility stimulant

3 (a) **True**   Glomerular filtration rate decreases approximately 10
  (b) **True**   mL/min for every decade over 30, i.e. decreases with age.
  (c) **True**   See *TCP*, Chapter 11, p. 78. Dalteparin is a low molecular
  (d) **True**   weight heparin.
  (e) **True**

4 The metabolism of the following drugs can be saturated within the usual dose range:

   (a) Morphine
   (b) Tobramycin
   (c) Heparin
   (d) Ethanol (alcohol)
   (e) Phenytoin

5 The elimination half-life of the following drugs is greater than 12 hours:

   (a) Heparin
   (b) Adenosine
   (c) Diazepam
   (d) Fluoxetine
   (e) Azithromycin

6 The following drugs block re-uptake of 5-hydroxytryptamine:

   (a) Buspirone
   (b) Dextromethorphan
   (c) Pizotifen
   (d) Granisetron
   (e) Paroxetine

7 Individuals who are categorized as slow acetylators (i.e. have a relatively low activity of hepatic N-acetyltransferase):

   (a) Have a prevalence of 15–20% in European Caucasians
   (b) Are more likely to develop thrombocytopenia, nephrotic syndrome and rash during gold treatment
   (c) Are more likely to develop hepatotoxicity following halothane anesthesia
   (d) Are more likely to develop antinuclear antibodies during hydralazine therapy
   (e) Are more likely to develop peripheral neuropathy during isoniazid therapy

4 (a) **False**   For drugs that exhibit saturation kinetics a small increase in
   (b) **False**   dose can lead to a disproportionate increase in plasma
   (c) **True**   concentration.
   (d) **True**
   (e) **True**

5 (a) **False** – 0.5–2.5 hours
   (b) **False** – 5–10 seconds
   (c) **True** – Approximately 36–48 hours
   (d) **True** – Approximately 48 hours
   (e) **True** – Approximately 68 hours

6 (a) **False** – Partial agonist
   (b) **True** – If taken with MAO-I or SSRI could produce coma, rigidity,
                   myoclonus – "serotonin syndrome"
   (c) **False** – 5-HT$_{1+2}$ antagonist (migraine prophylaxis)
   (d) **False** – 5-HT$_3$ antagonist
   (e) **True** – SSRI antidepressant

7 (a) **False**
   (b) **False**
   (c) **False**
   (d) **True**
   (e) **True**

Table 8 Variations in drug metabolism due to some genetic polymorphisms

Pharmacogenetic variation	Mechanism	Inheritance	Occurrence	Drugs involved
Rapid acetylator status	Increased hepatic N-acetyltransferase	Autosomal dominant	40% whites	Isoniazid; hydralazine; some phenelzine; dapsone; procainamide
Suxamethonium sensitivity	Several types of abnormal plasma pseudocholinesterase	Autosomal recessive	Most common form 1:2500	Suxamethonium
Defective hydroxylation of debrisoquine	Functionally defective cytochrome CYP2D6	Autosomal recessive	8% Britons; 1% Saudi Arabians; 30% Chinese	Debrisoquine; metoprolol; perhexiline; nortriptyline
Ethanol sensitivity	Relatively low rate of alcohol metabolism	Usual in some ethnic groups	Orientals	Alcohol

8 The following drugs are believed to be teratogenic in man:

   (a) Phenytoin
   (b) Acitretin (retinoid)
   (c) Methotrexate
   (d) Warfarin
   (e) Ribavirin

9 Which of the following is generally suitable for the management of community acquired lower UTI diagnosed during pregnancy:

   (a) Amoxicillin
   (b) Cefadroxil
   (c) Oxytetracycline
   (d) Co-trimoxazole
   (e) Ciprofloxacin

10 SSRI antidepressants such as fluoxetine and sertraline:

   (a) Commonly cause anticholinergic side effects
   (b) Commonly cause postural hypotension
   (c) Commonly cause broadening of the QRS in overdose
   (d) Have been shown to be less effective in endogenous depression than older antidepressants such as amitriptyline
   (e) Should be stopped at least 2 weeks before electroconvulsive therapy

11 Carbidopa when combined with levodopa:

   (a) Inhibits the intracerebral metabolism of levodopa
   (b) Reduces nausea by permitting a lower dose of levodopa
   (c) Reduces postural hypotension by permitting a lower dose of levodopa
   (d) Delays the onset of improvement in bradykinesia
   (e) Abolishes the "on-off" phenomenon

12 Carbamazepine:

   (a) Is structurally related to the tricyclic antidepressants
   (b) Induces its own metabolism via hepatic CYP3A
   (c) Increases chloride conductance at the $GABA_A$ receptor
   (d) Is contraindicated in patients with hypertrophic obstructive cardiomyopathy
   (e) May cause hyponatremia

8 (a) **True**
  (b) **True**
  (c) **True**
  (d) **True**
  (e) **True**

Table 9 Some drugs that are definitely teratogenic

Thalidomide	Androgens
Cytotoxic agents	Progestogens
Ethanol (alcohol)	Ribavirin
Warfarin	Radioisotopes
Retinoids	Some live vaccines
Most anticonvulsants	Lithium

Some drugs, e.g. misoprostol, ergotamine, can cause abortion.

9 (a) **True**   Urinary tract infection in pregnancy should be treated
  (b) **True**   without delay to prevent progression to pyelonephritis.
  (c) **False**
  (d) **False**
  (e) **False**

10 (a) **False**   SSRIs are less toxic in overdose, and associated with fewer and
   (b) **False**   generally less severe adverse effects than tricyclic
   (c) **False**   antidepressants. They are now regarded by many as first line
   (d) **False**   treatment in most patients with endogenous depression.
   (e) **False**

11 (a) **False**   Carbidopa, a peripheral dopa decarboxylase inhibitor,
   (b) **True**   inhibits the extracerebral metabolism of the levodopa to
   (c) **True**   dopamine.
   (d) **False**
   (e) **False**

12 (a) **True**   Carbamazepine is an anticonvulsant which is also sometimes
   (b) **True**   used in the treatment of diabetes insipidus, painful diabetic
   (c) **False**   neuropathy, post-herpetic neuralgia and trigeminal
   (d) **False**   neuralgia.
   (e) **True**

13 It is rational and advised therapeutic practice to commence treatment with the following drugs using a loading dose if a rapid onset of action is required:

(a) Digoxin
(b) Zolmitriptan
(c) Amiodarone
(d) Levodopa
(e) Phenytoin

14 Enalapril has the following properties:

(a) Inhibits conversion of renin to angiotensin
(b) Inhibits the degradation of bradykinin
(c) Increases urinary elimination of potassium
(d) Can be used as a mixed arterial and venous dilator in heart failure
(e) Is safe in pregnancy

15 A man is admitted within 3 hours of the onset of chest pain. His ECG is consistent with an acute myocardial infarction. Streptokinase should not be administered if:

(a) The patient is over 70 years old
(b) The patient had a stroke due to a cerebral hemorrhage 3 months previously
(c) The patient is already taking atenolol for hypertension (average blood pressure on treatment of 150/95)
(d) The patient has asthma
(e) The patient received streptokinase 3 months previously following a myocardial infarction

16 The following agents may be used in the long-term treatment of chronic atrial fibrillation in a 55-year-old female:

(a) Mexiletine
(b) Warfarin
(c) Adenosine
(d) Sotalol
(e) Digoxin

13 (a) **True** It takes approximately five times the half-life to reach steady
   (b) **False** state plasma concentrations. A loading dose is rational for a
   (c) **True** drug with a long half-life if a rapid onset of action is
   (d) **False** required, the effect is related to plasma concentration and
   (e) **True** administering the loading dose is safe.

14 (a) **False** – Inhibits angiotensin I conversion to angiotensin II
   (b) **True** – May be the cause of cough in up to 30% of patients
   (c) **False** – Can cause hyperkalemia
   (d) **True**
   (e) **False**

15 (a) **False** – Even greater reduction in mortality
   (b) **True**
   (c) **False**
   (d) **False**
   (e) **True** – Give recombinant tissue plasminogen activator (r-tpa)

16 (a) **False** – A class 1 antiarrhythmic drug
   (b) **True** – Reduces the risk of embolism
   (c) **False** – Used in the diagnosis and immediate treatment of SVT
   (d) **True** – A β-blocker with additional class III antiarrhythmic activity
   (e) **True** – Cardiac glycosides are especially useful for controlling
              ventricular response in atrial fibrillation by reducing
              conduction in the AV node

17 Estimation of plasma/serum drug concentrations are useful in optimizing the therapeutic dose required of:

(a) Warfarin
(b) Omeprazole
(c) Lithium carbonate
(d) Risperidone
(e) Cyclosporin

18 The following antiarrhythmic treatments are correctly paired with an appropriate indication:

(a) Digoxin – rapid atrial fibrillation
(b) Verapamil – atrial fibrillation complicating WPW
(c) Lignocaine – ventricular arrhythmias post-myocardial infarction
(d) Atropine – symptomatic bradycardia post-myocardial infarction
(e) Demand atrio-ventricular pacemaker – first degree heart block

19 Enoxaparin

(a) Is absolutely contraindicated in pregnancy
(b) Is monitored by measurement of the activated partial thromboplastin time (APTT)
(c) Is much less effective in patients with protein C deficiency
(d) Is reversed by vitamin K
(e) Has a shorter duration of action than heparin

20 The following agents are associated with a decreased clearance of theophylline:

(a) St John's wort
(b) Erythromycin
(c) Ciprofloxacin
(d) Phenytoin
(e) Rifampicin

21 The following are indicated in acute severe asthma in a boy of 12 years:

(a) High inspired oxygen concentration (Fio_2 of 40%)
(b) Nebulized salbutamol
(c) Intravenous hydrocortisone
(d) Intravenous isoprenaline
(e) Oral montelukast

17 (a) **False** – Warfarin concentrations are rarely if ever measured. Monitor the pharmacodynamic effect on prothrombin time.
   (b) **False** – Omeprazole inhibits gastric acid production
   (c) **True** – In addition to serum concentrations thyroid function should be monitored
   (d) **False** – Risperidone is used to treat schizophrenia. Cardiac arrhythmias have been reported and an ECG should be performed before starting therapy and periodically afterwards at doses over 8 mg daily
   (e) **True** – Cyclosporin is a potent immunosuppressant which is of particular value in organ transplantation. It has little effect on the bone marrow but is nephrotoxic. There is considerable interindividual variability in its pharmacokinetics

18 (a) **True** – NB: cardioversion is often effective in acute AF
   (b) **False** – May increase ventricular rate
   (c) **True**
   (d) **True**
   (e) **False** – No therapy indicated

19 (a) **False** – Is used in management of thromboembolic disease in pregnancy
   (b) **False** – If monitoring is required (rare) measure anti-Xa activity in plasma
   (c) **False** – Antagonism of factor Xa is its major site of action
   (d) **False** – Can be reversed with protamine, 1 mg protamine per 1 mg of enoxaparin
   (e) **False** – For most indications, once daily administration is satisfactory

20 (a) **False**   Theophylline is metabolized by CYP_{4501A2}, St John's wort.
   (b) **True**   Phenytoin and rifampicin induce CYP_{4501A2} (as does
   (c) **True**   smoking) whilst erythromycin and ciprofloxacin inhibit
   (d) **False** CYP_{4501A2}. Theophylline has a narrow therapeutic index
   (e) **False**   hence such interactions are clinically significant.

21 (a) **True**   The increasing mortality of acute severe asthma is partially
   (b) **True**   due to failure to recognize the severity of an exacerbation
   (c) **True**   and delayed initiation of treatment with glucocorticosteroids.
   (d) **False**
   (e) **False** – Oral leukotriene antagonists are not of proven efficacy in acute severe asthma

22 The following drugs reduce gastric acid secretion:

(a) Sucralfate
(b) Ranitidine
(c) Pantoprazole
(d) Loperamide
(e) Bismuth

23 Lansoprazole:

(a) Inhibits the hydrogen–potassium adenosine triphosphatase enzyme system
(b) Is a synthetic analog of prostaglandin E_2
(c) Blackens the tongue
(d) Is an effective treatment for peptic ulcer associated with *H. pylori*
(e) Is effective in treating reflux esophagitis

24 The following are associated with dose-dependent hepatotoxicity:

(a) Paracetamol (acetaminophen)
(b) Halothane
(c) Methotrexate
(d) Azathioprine
(e) Erythromycin lactobionate

22 (a) **False** – A complex of aluminum hydroxide and sulfated sucrose
   (b) **True** – An H$_2$-blocker
   (c) **True** – A proton pump inhibitor like omeprazole, lansoprazole, etc.
   (d) **False** – An anti-motility drug used as an adjunct to fluid and electrolyte replacement in diarrhea
   (e) **False** – Stimulates mucosal protective prostaglandin, bicarbonate secretion and has a direct toxic effect on *Helicobacter pylori*

23 (a) **True**
   (b) **False** – Misoprostol is a synthetic prostaglandin analog
   (c) **False** – Bismuth blackens the tongue
   (d) **True**
   (e) **True**

24 (a) **True**
   (b) **False**
   (c) **True**
   (d) **True**
   (e) **False**

Table 10 Dose-dependent hepatotoxicity

Drug	Mechanism	Comment/predisposing factors
Paracetamol	Hepatitis	See Chapter 53 (*TCP*)
Salicylates	Focal hepatocellular necrosis	Autoimmune disease (especially SLE)
	Reye's syndrome	In children – viral infection
Tetracycline	Central and mid-zonal necrosis with fat droplets	
Azathioprine	Cholestasis + hepatitis	Underlying liver disease
Methotrexate	Hepatic fibrosis	
Fusidic acid	Cholestasis, conjugated hyperbilirubinemi(a)	Rare
Rifampicin	Cholestasis, mixed conjugated and unconjugated hyperbilirubinemia	Transient
Synthetic estrogens	Cholestasis, may precipitate gall stones	Underlying liver disease rare now low-dose estrogens are generally given
HMGCoA reductase inhibitors	Unknown	Usually mild and asymptomatic

SLE Systemic lupus erythematosus.

25 The following drugs should be avoided in patients with liver disease who are jaundiced with ascites:

   (a) Diazepam
   (b) Spironolactone
   (c) Magnesium trisilicate mixture
   (d) Indomethacin
   (e) Metronidazole

26 Calcipotriol:

   (a) Is indicated in plaque psoriasis
   (b) Is a derivative of vitamin D
   (c) Causes marked erythema if applied to normal skin
   (d) Causes yellow discoloration of the skin but not sclerae
   (e) May cause hypercalcemia

27 The following treatment is appropriate for the indication named:

   (a) Cellulitis – phenoxymethyl penicillin and flucloxacillin
   (b) Typhoid fever – ciprofloxacin
   (c) Meningococcal meningitis – benzylpenicillin
   (d) Herpes simplex encephalitis – acyclovir
   (e) Threadworm infection in a child > 2 years – mebendazole

28 Treatment with intravenous gentamicin:

   (a) Is contraindicated in neonatal septicemia
   (b) Is effectively given as a once daily administered dose
   (c) Is relatively contraindicated in myasthenia gravis
   (d) Is associated with ototoxicity which is usually irreversible
   (e) Is contraindicated in cystic fibrosis patients with an exacerbation of their respiratory disease

29 The following drugs have been correctly paired with an associated severe adverse effect:

   (a) Cisplatin – nausea and vomiting
   (b) Omeprazole – gastric carcinoma
   (c) Clindamycin – pseudomembranous colitis
   (d) Interferon-α – Kaposi's sarcoma
   (e) Doxorubicin – cardiomyopathy

25 (a) **True** – Long $t\frac{1}{2}$. Active metabolite. Can precipitate coma
   (b) **False** – Aldosterone antagonist useful in treatment of edema in hepatic failure
   (c) **False**
   (d) **True** – Increased risk of gastrointestinal bleeding and fluid retention
   (e) **False**

26 (a) **True**
   (b) **True**
   (c) **False** – Unlike dithranol
   (d) **False** – Unlike β-carotene
   (e) **True** – Reported if recommended dose exceeded or when applied to generalized pustular or erythrodermic exfoliative psoriasis

27 (a) **True** – Co-amoxiclav is an alternative. If the patient is penicillin-allergic, erythromycin may be used. If severe, parenteral antibiotics may be necessary
   (b) **True** – Chloramphenicol is also effective
   (c) **True** – Cefotaxime is also effective and penetrates CSF well
   (d) **True**
   (e) **True** – Mebendazole is also effective in hookworm and roundworm infections

28 (a) **False**   The aminoglycosides are effective in some Gram-positive and
   (b) **True**   many Gram-negative infections. They are not absorbed from
   (c) **True**   the gut, are principally eliminated in the urine and have a
   (d) **True**   low therapeutic ratio. Plasma drug concentrations should be
   (e) **False**   monitored. Once daily therapy is being used more widely.

29 (a) **True** – May be reduced by $5HT_3$ antagonists e.g. ondansetron or high dose metoclopramide
   (b) **False**
   (c) **True** – Treated with oral vancomycin or metronidazole
   (d) **False** – Used to treat AIDS-related Kaposi's sarcoma
   (e) **True** – Associated with cumulative dose when standard treatment regimens are used

30 The first line treatment of pulmonary TB in a UK native who is immunocompetent includes an initial phase of 2 months treatment with:

  (a) Isoniazid
  (b) Rifampicin
  (c) Pyrazinamide
  (d) Ethambutol
  (e) Streptomycin

31 A 25-year-old pregnant woman who was using chloroquine as malaria prophylaxis returns to the UK with cerebral malaria. The woman is 27 weeks pregnant. The following are appropriate:

  (a) Immediate delivery of the fetus
  (b) Intravenous quinine
  (c) Intravenous quinine and intravenous chloroquine in combination
  (d) Intravenous dexamethasone
  (e) The patient should be tested for G6PDH deficiency before starting the treatment

32 The following are likely to be useful in reducing the plasma calcium concentration in a patient with severe hypercalcemia associated with myeloma:

  (a) Intravenous 0.9% saline
  (b) Methylprednisolone
  (c) Hydrochlorothiazide
  (d) Calcitonin
  (e) Disodium pamidronate

33 The following may be effective in the management of oral candidiasis:

  (a) Nystatin
  (b) Doxycycline
  (c) Amphotericin
  (d) Fluconazole
  (e) Valciclovir

30 (a) **True**   Ethambutol and/or streptomycin are included in a 4 drug
   (b) **True**   regimen if resistance is suspected, predicted or known.
   (c) **True**
   (d) **False**
   (e) **False**

31 (a) **False**   Cerebral malaria has a particularly high morbidity/mortality
   (b) **True**   in pregnancy. Quinine is life-saving and must be initiated as
   (c) **False**   soon as possible.
   (d) **True**   Steroids reduce cerebral complications
   (e) **False**

32 (a) **True**   Severe hypercalcemia is a medical emergency. Initial and
   (b) **True**   immediate rehydration is essential.
   (c) **False**   Thiazides reduce renal calcium clearance
   (d) **True**
   (e) **True**

33 (a) **True**   Broad-spectrum antibiotics, diabetes, inhaled steroids and
   (b) **False**   immunosuppression are predisposing factors in the
   (c) **True**   development of oral candidiasis.
   (d) **True**
   (e) **False**

34 Human insulin:

(a) Is usually produced from highly purified human pancreas
(b) Inhibits the subjective awareness of hypoglycemia
(c) Should not be given intravenously
(d) Is considerably more expensive than porcine insulin
(e) Should not be given concurrently with lisinopril

35 Allopurinol:

(a) Increases urinary elimination of uric acid
(b) Inhibits leukocyte migration
(c) Inhibits xanthine oxidase
(d) Reduces the plasma uric acid
(e) Should not be prescribed concurrently with a non-steroidal anti-inflammatory drug (NSAID)

36 The following drugs should be avoided in severe renal impairment:

(a) Capecitabine
(b) Oxytetracycline
(c) Metolazone
(d) Metformin
(e) Fybogel

37 The following drugs are correctly paired with their putative mode of action:

(a) Ondansetron – $5HT_3$ receptor antagonist
(b) Ropinirole – dopamine D_2 receptor agonist
(c) Rofecoxib – blockade of platelet glycoprotein IIb/IIIa receptors
(d) Olanzapine – $5HT_2$ receptor agonist
(e) Sildenafil – inhibition of tissue necrosis factor (TNF)

38 A 16-year-old girl develops acute angioedema with stridor following an injection of intravenous ampicillin in the casualty department. The following are indicated:

(a) Immediate intramuscular adrenaline
(b) Intravenous serum C1q esterase inhibitor
(c) Intravenous metoclopramide
(d) Inhaled theophylline
(e) In addition to ampicillin, clarithromycin should be avoided in the future

34 (a) **False**   Human insulin can now be produced by recombinant
   (b) **False**   technology and is routinely used in newly diagnosed insulin
   (c) **False**   dependent diabetics.
   (d) **False**
   (e) **False**

35 (a) **False**   Allopurinol is used prophylactically in the management of
   (b) **False**   gout. When allopurinol is started it may precipitate an acute
   (c) **True**   attack, hence it should be prescribed with an NSAID initially.
   (d) **True**
   (e) **False**

36 (a) **True** – Accumulates and causes increased bone marrow toxicity
   (b) **True** – Antianabolic effect, increases urea, impairs renal function
   (c) **False**
   (d) **True** – Increased risk of lactic acidosis
   (e) **True** – Contains 7 mmol potassium per sachet

37 (a) **True** – Particularly valuable in preventing cisplatin induced
        vomiting
   (b) **True** – Used in Parkinson's disease
   (c) **False** – Rofecoxib and celecoxib are selective cyclo-oxygenase 2
        inhibitors. Eptifibiatide and tirofiban inhibit platelet
        aggregation by binding to platelet glycoprotein IIb/IIIa
        receptors
   (d) **False** – Olanzapine is an antagonist of $5HT_2$ receptors. It is also an
        antagonist at D4, D1, D2 and muscarinic receptors. LSD and
        other hallucinogens such as MDMA probably owe their
        hallucinogenic effect due to $5HT_2$-agonist properties
   (e) **False** – Sildenafil is a phosphodieterase (PDE5) inhibitor. Infliximab
        (a monoclonal antibody) inhibits TNF activity. It is used in
        Crohn's disease and rheumatoid arthritis unresponsive to
        more established therapies

38 (a) **True**   In addition to intramuscular adrenaline, oxygen, intravenous
   (b) **False** corticosteroids, intravenous fluids and intravenous
   (c) **False** antihistamine are usually administered.
   (d) **False**
   (e) **False**

39 The following drugs may cause gynecomastia:

(a) Spironolactone
(b) Riluzole
(c) Cimetidine
(d) Flupentixol (flupenthixol)
(e) Ketoconazole

40 A 20-year-old girl is admitted to the casualty department unconscious. There is reliable circumstantial evidence that she ingested 50 of her grandmother's amitriptyline tablets and 50 quinine tablets within the last hour. On admission, in addition to a grade IV coma, she has dilated pupils and brisk reflexes. Her blood pressure is 100/60, pulse 100 bpm. She is not cyanosed. Minute volumes and blood gases are acceptable. The ECG shows a wide QRS with prolonged QTc. The following are appropriate:

(a) ECG monitoring
(b) Stomach washout following placement of a cuffed endotracheal tube
(c) Intravenous disopyramide
(d) Forced acid diuresis
(e) Stellate ganglion block to prevent blindness

41 A 14-year-old girl is seen in the A & E department. She is complaining of tinnitus and is hyperventilating and admits to having ingested a variety of at least 50 tablets from her parents' medicine cupboard, approximately 7 hours ago. The following statements are true:

(a) Blood should be taken for salicylate concentration
(b) Blood should be taken for paracetamol concentration
(c) Blood should be taken for fluoxetine concentrations
(d) Blood should be taken for morphine concentrations
(e) An arterial sample should be taken for pH and blood gas estimation

42 The management of a thyrotoxic crisis ("thyroid storm") usually requires treatment with:

(a) Intravenous fluids
(b) Propranolol
(c) Hydrocortisone
(d) Radioiodine I^{131}
(e) Propylthiouracil

39 (a) **True**   Riluzole is used to extend life or the time to mechanical
   (b) **False** ventilation in patients with motor neuron disease who have
   (c) **True**   amyotrophic lateral sclerosis.
   (d) **True**
   (e) **True**

40 (a) **True**   Tricyclic antidepressants have a high mortality in overdose.
   (b) **True**   In addition to cardiac arrhythmias, convulsions are a recog-
   (c) **False** nized potentially fatal complication.
   (d) **False**
   (e) **False**

41 (a) **True**   Patients who have taken a significant salicylate overdose
   (b) **True**   commonly present hyperventilating and complaining of
   (c) **False** tinnitus. If there is any possibility of paracetamol overdose,
   (d) **False** its plasma concentration should be measured as effective
   (e) **True**   antidotes are available.

42 (a) **True**   Thyrotoxic crisis requires emergency treatment. Carbimazole
   (b) **True**   or propylthiouracil may be administered by nasogastric tube
   (c) **True**   if the oral route is impractical. Propylthiouracil may be
   (d) **False** preferred in "thyroid storm" because of its additional
   (e) **True**   peripheral action blocking conversion of T4 to T3. The
   hydrocortisone and propranolol are usually given by
   intravenous injection.

43 The following drugs cause constipation:

(a) Verapamil
(b) Dihydrocodeine
(c) Ondansetron
(d) Misoprostol
(e) Antacids containing aluminum

44 The combined oral contraceptive should not be prescribed if:

(a) There is a history of severe or focal migraine
(b) The girl is aged 16 and her parents have not consented
(c) There is a history of deep vein thrombosis
(d) Major elective surgery is planned within 4 weeks
(e) There is a history of porphyria

45 Hormone replacement therapy is contraindicated if there is a history of:

(a) Depression
(b) Breast cancer
(c) Hysterectome
(d) Chronic obstructive bronchitis
(e) Eczema

46 The following drugs are nephrotoxic:

(a) Fluconazole
(b) Atorvastatin
(c) Amikacin
(d) Amphotericin B
(e) Tacrolimus (FK 506)

47 The following drugs may precipitate bronchospasm:

(a) Ibuprofen
(b) Codeine phosphate
(c) Labetalol
(d) Aspirin
(e) Adenosine

43 (a) **True**
   (b) **True**
   (c) **True**
   (d) **False**
   (e) **True**

44 (a) **True**   The combined oral contraceptive should also be avoided
   (b) **False**   if there is undiagnosed vaginal bleeding, genital
   (c) **True**   carcinoma, liver disease, valvular heart disease or a
   (d) **True**   history of arterial embolism.
   (e) **True**

45 (a) **False**   In addition to preventing menopausal vasomotor
   (b) **True**   symptoms and menopausal vaginitis if small doses of
   (c) **False**   estrogen are started in the perimenopausal period the
   (d) **False**   incidence of osteoporosis, stroke and myocardial
   (e) **False**   infarction are reduced. Unless the patient has had a
               hysterectomy, a cyclic progestogen must be used to prevent
               the increased risk of endometrial cancer.

46 (a) **False** – An azole anti-fungal
   (b) **False** – An HMGCoA reductase inhibitor
   (c) **True** – Monitoring of aminoglycoside concentrations is mandatory
                 in renal impairment.
   (d) **True** – An antifungal agent often required in renal disease due to
                 immunosuppression
   (e) **True** – An immunosuppressant used in the management of solid
                 organ transplantation

47 (a) **True** – All NSAIDs can precipitate bronchospasm in susceptible
                 asthmatics
   (b) **True** – Opioids can precipitate bronchospasm
   (c) **True** – A combined α- and β-blocker (β-blocking effects
                 predominate)
   (d) **True**
   (e) **True** – Used in diagnosis/treatment of SVT

48 Non-steroidal anti-inflammatory drugs:

(a) Reduce the effectiveness of loop diuretics
(b) Reduce glomerular filtration in patients with glomerulonephritis
(c) Impair the renal excretion of lithium
(d) Are recognized causes of acute interstitial nephritis
(e) Significantly increase urinary excretion of PGE_2

49 The following drugs are correctly paired with a recognized unwanted effect:

(a) Vincristine and peripheral neuropathy
(b) Nifedipine and peripheral edema
(c) Trastuzumab and anaphylaxis
(d) Metoclopramide and oculogyric crisis
(e) Bleomycin and pulmonary fibrosis

50 Drug-induced hyperkalemia may be caused by:

(a) Amiloride
(b) Spironolactone
(c) Chronic laxative treatment
(d) High dose trimethoprim/sulfamethoxazole
(e) Heparin

51 Erythromycin:

(a) Penetrates the CSF well
(b) Is effective in *Mycoplasma* pneumonia
(c) Inhibits cytochrome P_{450}
(d) Is concentrated in the urine
(e) Is effective in non-specific urethritis

52 The following drugs may be used in acute porphyria for an appropriate indication:

(a) Quinine
(b) Atenolol
(c) Oral contraceptive agents
(d) Heparin
(e) Amoxycillin

48 (a) **True**   NSAIDs should be avoided if possible in renal disease.
   (b) **True**   The advantages of low dose aspirin in myocardial
   (c) **True**   infarction and unstable angina generally outweigh any
   (d) **True**   disadvantages.
   (e) **False**

49 (a) **True**
   (b) **True**   – Largely unresponsive to diuretics
   (c) **True**   – Monoclonal antibody for metastatic breast cancer in patients
             whose tumors over-express the human epidermal growth
             receptor 2 (HER2)
   (d) **True**   – Treated with diazepam or an anticholinergic such as
             benztropine
   (e) **True**

50 (a) **True**   Drug-induced hyperkalemia is particularly dangerous if there
   (b) **True**   is impaired renal function. The emergency treatment
   (c) **False** includes intravenous calcium chloride, intravenous glucose
   (d) **True**   and insulin, sodium bicarbonate. To increase the elimination
   (e) **True**   of potassium, calcium resonium and/or
             hemofiltration/hemodialysis are effective.

51 (a) **False** Erythromycin is a macrolide antibiotic. It is a useful
   (b) **True**   alternative to penicillin but is no use in meningitis.
   (c) **True**   Erythromycin is also effective against chlamydia, legionella,
   (d) **False** mycoplasma and campylobacter.
   (e) **True**

52 (a) **True**   Acute illness is precipitated by drugs because of inherited
   (b) **True**   enzyme deficiencies in the pathway of heme synthesis. Drug-
   (c) **False** induced exacerbations of acute porphyria (neurological,
   (d) **True**   psychiatric, cardiovascular and gastrointestinal disturbances
   (e) **True**   that are occasionally fatal) are accompanied by increased
             urinary excretion of 5-aminolevulinic acid (ALA) and
             porphobilinogen.

53 The following drugs cause pupillary constriction (miosis):

(a) Dextropropoxyphene
(b) Neostigmine
(c) Amitriptyline
(d) Salmeterol
(e) Pilocarpine eye drops

54 Adverse effects associated with zidovudine (AZT) include:

(a) Neutrophilia
(b) Nausea and vomiting
(c) Mitochondrial myopathy
(d) Anemia
(e) Nephrotic syndrome

55 In the use of anti-retroviral therapy for HIV infection the following statements are true:

(a) Zalcitabine (ddC) causes a peripheral neuropathy
(b) The myopathy induced by AZT is irreversible
(c) The HIV protease inhibitor, indinavir, causes renal stones
(d) Ritonavir induces the metabolism of drugs metabolized by CYP3A4
(e) The combination of AZT or ddI and d4T (stavudine) may be synergistic against HIV proliferation

56 The following drugs are associated with a facial "butterfly" rash:

(a) Ranitidine
(b) Phenytoin
(c) Lisinopril
(d) Isoniazid
(e) Hydralazine

57 The following drugs exert their therapeutic action by inhibition of the paired named enzyme:

(a) Vigabatrin – GABA transaminase
(b) Selegiline – dopa decarboxylase
(c) Moclobemide – monoamine oxidase A
(d) Foscarnet – RNA transcriptase
(e) Enalaprilat – angiotension converting enzyme

53 (a) **True**   Pupil constriction is a sign of opioid overdose. Cholino-
   (b) **True**   mimetics also cause miosis as does pontine hemorrhage. If
   (c) **False**   there is asymmetry an intracerebral space occupying lesion
   (d) **False**   (e.g. hematoma) or local lesion should be considered.
   (e) **True**

54 (a) **False**   AZT does not cure AIDS but may delay its progression. It has
   (b) **True**   a characteristic toxicity profile including anemia and
   (c) **True**   neutropenia.
   (d) **True**
   (e) **False**

55 (a) **True**
   (b) **False** – Myopathy improves on drug withdrawal
   (c) **True**
   (d) **False** – Ritonavir (and most other HIV protease inhibitors) inhibits
                    CYP3A4 drug metabolism
   (e) **False** – *In vitro* data suggest antagonism of this combination – thus
                    these combinations are avoided in clinical use

56 (a) **False**   Drug-induced SLE is usually reversible on withdrawing the
   (b) **True**   causative drug. It tends not to affect the kidneys.
   (c) **False**
   (d) **True**
   (e) **True**

57 (a) **True**
   (b) **False** – Inhibits MAO-B
   (c) **True**
   (d) **False** – Foscarnet is a pyrophosphate (triphosphate analog) and
                    competitive inhibitor of DNA polymerase
   (e) **True**

58 The following drugs may cause or exacerbate hypercalcaemia:

   (a) Bendrofluazide
   (b) Frusemide (furosemide)
   (c) Dexamethasone
   (d) Calcium resonium
   (e) 1-α-Hydroxycholecalciferol

59 The following are recognized causes of neutropenia:

   (a) 6-Mercaptopurine
   (b) Penicillamine
   (c) Carbamazepine
   (d) Clozapine
   (e) Paclitaxel

60 A 60-year-old man with a history of gout, diabetes and mild asthma (not requiring regular medication) is diagnosed as having essential hypertension. Which of the following drugs might be suitable?

   (a) Hydrochlorothiazide
   (b) Atenolol
   (c) Diltiazem controlled release
   (d) Trandolapril
   (e) Doxazosin

58 (a) **True** – A thiazide diuretic
   (b) **False** – A loop diuretic
   (c) **False** – A corticosteroid
   (d) **True** – An ion exchange resin used to remove excess potassium
   (e) **True** – A vitamin D derivative and precursor of 1,25-dihydroxychole-calciferol which may cause or exacerbate hypercalcemia

59 (a) **True**   Early appropriate drug withdrawal reduces the morbidity/
   (b) **True**   mortality. Granulocyte colony-stimulating factor (G-CSF) is
   (c) **True**   sometimes effective in the management of drug-induced
   (d) **True**   myelosuppression.
   (e) **True**

60 (a) **False** – Increases plasma urate and impairs glucose tolerance
   (b) **False** – Contraindicated in asthma. Whilst not contraindicated in
       diabetes, β-blockers should be avoided in patients with
       hypoglycemic episodes as they interfere with the metabolic
       and autonomic responses to hypoglycemia. The latter effect
       masks the warning symptoms and signs of hypoglycemia
   (c) **True**
   (d) **True** – ACE inhibitors reduce risk of renal deterioration in diabetes
   (e) **True**

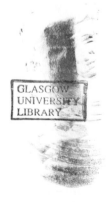
GLASGOW
UNIVERSITY
LIBRARY